THE
Arthritis Foundation's
guide to
Alternative
THERAPIES

ARTHRITIS
FOUNDATION®

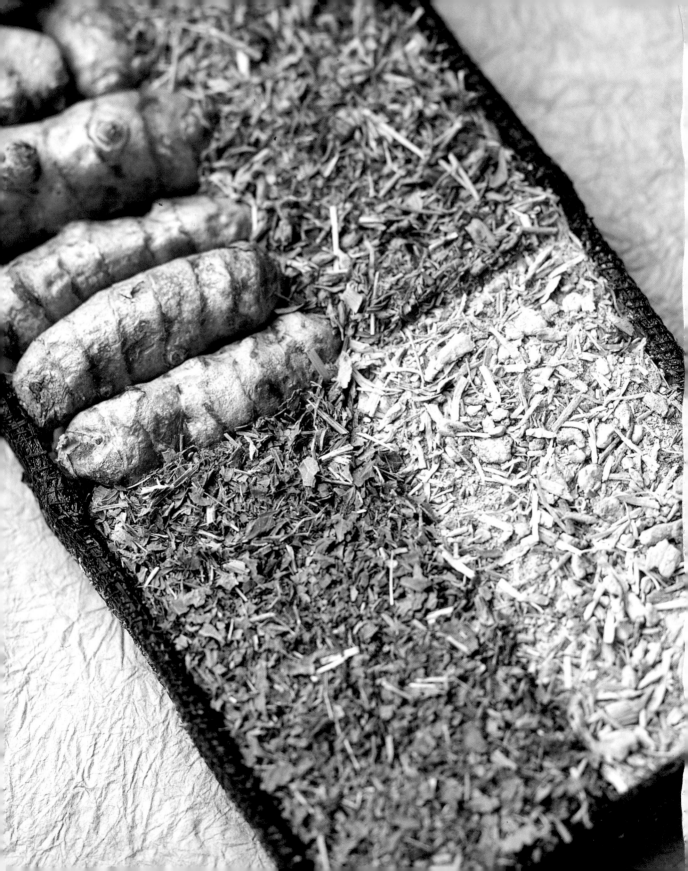

THE
Arthritis Foundation's
guide to
Alternative
THERAPIES

JUDITH HORSTMAN

Chief Medical Editor
William J. Arnold, MD

Associate Medical Editors
Brian Berman, MD
J. Roger Hollister, MD
Matthew H. Liang, MD, MPH

ARTHRITIS
FOUNDATION®

AN OFFICIAL PUBLICATION
OF THE ARTHRITIS FOUNDATION

Copyright 1999

Arthritis Foundation

1330 West Peachtree Street

Atlanta, GA 30309

Library of Congress Catalog Card Number: 99-61806

ISBN: 0-912423-23-4

Printed in Canada

———————————

This book was conceived, designed and
produced by the Arthritis Foundation

Editorial Director: ELIZABETH AXTELL

Art Director: AUDREY GRAHAM

Original Photography: PELOSI & CHAMBERS
Origianl Art: KATHRYN BORN

AUTHOR

Judith Horstman

Judith Horstman is an award-winning journalist who writes about health and medicine for doctors as well as the general public. A contributing editor for *Arthritis Today* magazine, her work has appeared in hundreds of publications including the *Harvard Health Letter*, *Hippocrates* and *USA Today*. She was a senior editor of *The Self-Care Advisor*, a family health guide, and edits a Web site for doctors on ALS (Lou Gehrig's Disease). She has also been a Washington correspondent, a journalism professor, and was the recipient of a Knight Science Journalism fellowship at MIT and two Fulbright Scholar grants. Ms. Horstman has practiced meditation and yoga for more than 25 years.

CHIEF MEDICAL EDITOR

William J. Arnold, MD, FACP, FACR

Executive Vice President and Medical Director
Advanced Bio-Surfaces, Inc.
Minnetonka, Minnesota

Dr. Bill Arnold is a practicing rheumatologist and the medical director of a company developing a new treatment option for osteoarthritis of the knee. Dr. Arnold graduated from the University of Illinois College of Medicine and completed his postgraduate training at Duke University. He is a member of the board of directors of the Park Ridge Center for Health, Faith and Ethics. He has been an active volunteer for the Arthritis Foundation for more than 20 years. Dr. Arnold's most recent appointment was to chair the Arthritis Foundation's Task Force on Complementary and Alternative Therapies. It was his role on the Task Force, as well as his interest in health, faith and ethics that brought him to edit this book.

ASSOCIATE MEDICAL EDITORS

Brian Berman, MD

Director
University of Maryland Complementary Medicine Program
Baltimore, Maryland

Dr. Brian Berman is Associate Professor of Family Medicine and founder and director of the University of Maryland Complementary Medicine Program, one of the first academic medical-based centers of research, education and clinical care in complementary medicine in the United States. He is board certified in family medicine and pain management. Dr. Berman has also trained extensively in acupuncture, homeopathy and other complementary therapies in the United States and abroad. He is principal investigator of a National Institutes of Health grant for alternative medicine research.

J. Roger Hollister, MD

Pediatric Rheumatology
The Children's Hospital
Denver, Colorado

Dr. Roger Hollister is Section Head, Pediatric Rheumatology at University of Colorado Health Sciences Center/The Children's Hospital in Denver. He has been treating children with rheumatic diseases and serving the community for 25 years. He has been a volunteer with the Arthritis Foundation, the American Juvenile Arthritis Organization and the Lupus Foundation. He currently is Chair, Complementary Therapies Subcommittee, Arthritis Foundation.

Matthew H. Liang, MD, MPH

Brigham and Women's Hospital
Boston, Massachusetts

Dr. Matt Liang is Professor of Medicine at Harvard Medical School and Professor of Health Policy and Management at Harvard School of Public Health. He is Director of the Robert B. Brigham Multipurpose Arthritis and Musculoskeletal Diseases Center and the Medical Director of Rehabilitation Services at Brigham and Women's Hospital. He directs the clinical research training program in rheumatology and is a member of the Brigham and Women's Hospital Research Institute's Clinical Research Committee. He is an active primary care physician and rheumatologist and has served on many Arthritis Foundation committees, including the Publishing Committee.

Contents

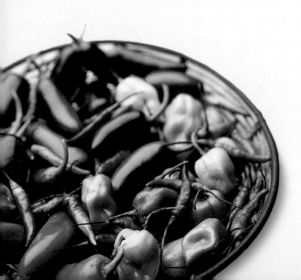

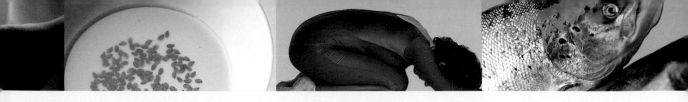

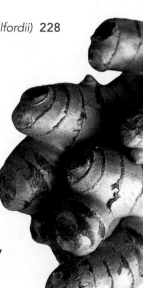

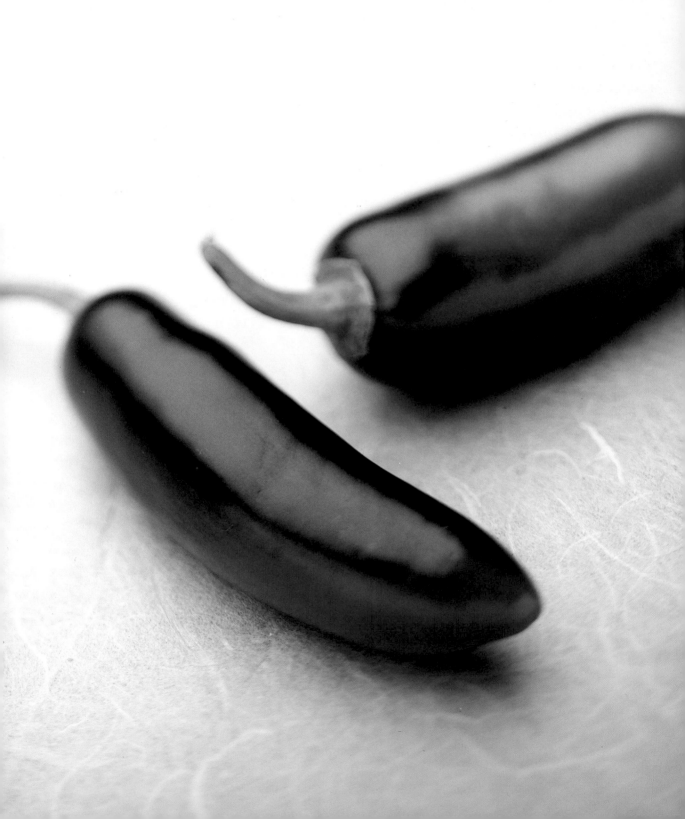

FOREWORD

Over the years, we at the Arthritis Foundation have been informing the public about research and treatments for arthritis. When it comes to unconventional therapies, the Foundation has often taken the path of warning you about the dangerous ones.

Recently, you have told us you want to know more. You've phoned, written and e-mailed us asking for information about complementary and alternative treatments that have promise, and not just warnings about which to avoid. You've told us, in no uncertain terms, that you are already using many of them, and want more information.

This book is a response to your questions and requests. We want to help you choose wisely and safely among the many therapies in the news. Many unconventional remedies may help you successfully manage your disease, especially when used along with your regular medical treatments. However, there are also "therapies" to approach with care. Our goal with this book is to lay the information down in front of you, not to tell you what to do. Read about a therapy, learn all that you can, and talk to your doctor before trying any new treatment.

We hope this book fulfills your needs. As more scientific evidence becomes available for unconventional therapies, look for a second volume.

ARTHRITIS FOUNDATION

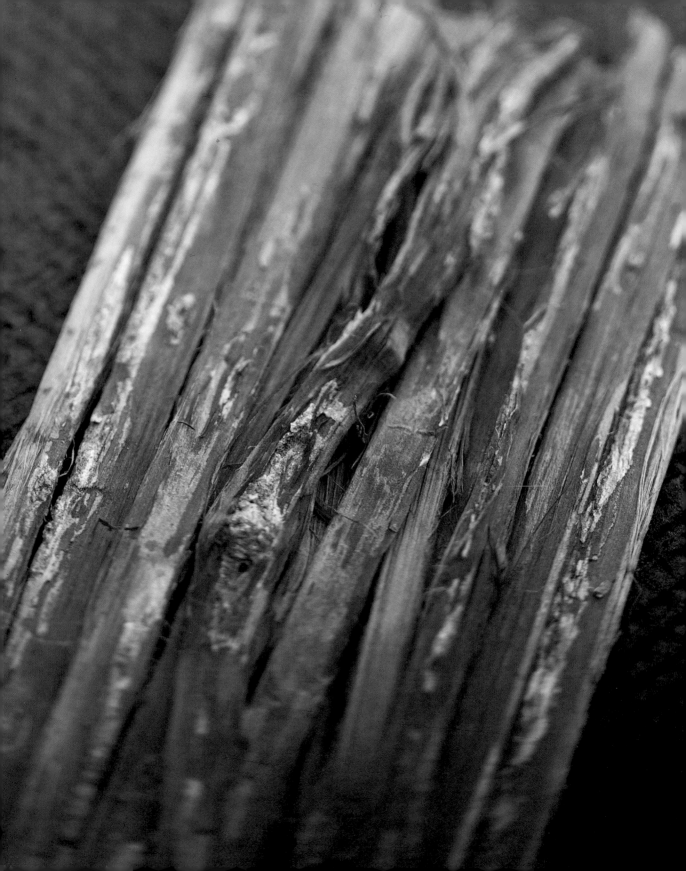

PROLOGUE

For every complex problem there is a simple answer –
and it is always wrong. — H.L. MENCKEN

Technology and the fascination of what it can accomplish is at the center of the psyche of Western scientists, physicians and the public at large. In our rush to find a "magic bullet" through technologic solutions, we have experienced a depersonalization of health care where the whole person is at risk of being lost in pursuit of a "cure." Thus, even though we have been gifted with the introduction of powerful new medications for arthritis, we need to abandon our "body-shop" approach for a more holistic perspective. Because there are no easy answers for the complex problems caused by arthritis, it is critical that people with arthritis and their physicians maintain a dialogue about the best approaches to treatment.

It is in this context that the issue of alternative therapies has come to the forefront. Their acceptance by many Americans is testament to their dissatisfaction with the present system of care. Alternative therapies provide people a sense of self-direction and control. Some of these treatments, however, fly in the face of accepted scientific principles and natural laws. When accompanied with aggressive and misleading marketing tactics that promise a "cure" for arthritis, many physicians automatically react negatively and refuse to discuss these therapies with their patients.

This book is part of the Arthritis Foundation's effort to bridge the gap between patients and their physicians by providing an unbiased source of information. The Foundation hopes to increase awareness of the risks and benefits of these treatments, as well as provide a common ground and encourage healthy dialogue between patients and physicians. This discourse will evolve and expand over time, depending on new research and the expressed needs of people with arthritis, their physicians and those who care both for and about them.

WILLIAM J. ARNOLD, MD

ACKNOWLEDGMENTS

The Arthritis Foundation gratefully acknowledges the following individuals and institutions for their assistance with this book. Their knowledge and insight make it a valuable resource for many people with arthritis and related conditions.

Arthritis Foundation Complementary Therapies Subcommittee

William J. Arnold, MD
Advanced Bio-Surfaces, Inc.
Minnetonka, Minn

Brian Berman, MD
Division of Complementary
  Medicine
University of Maryland
Baltimore, Md

Joan E. Broderick, PhD
Applied Behavioral Medical
  Research Institute
Department of Psychiatry
State University of New York at
  Stony Brook
Stony Brook, NY

Justus Fiechtner, MD
St. Lawrence Health Science Pavilion
East Lansing, Mich

Carol Henderson, PhD, RD
Epidemiologist/Registered Dietitian
Children's Hospital Medical Center
Cincinnati, Ohio

J. Roger Hollister, MD
Children's Hospital
Denver, Colo

Wayne B. Jonas, MD
Former Director
National Center for Complementary
  and Alternative Medicine
Bethesda, Md

Mayro Kanning
Patient Advocate
Cincinnati, Ohio

Richard Panush, MD
St. Barnabas Medical Center
Livingston, NJ

The following people reviewed chapters or provided information and insight

Laurence H. Altshuler, MD
Medical Director
Balanced Healing Medical Center
Oklahoma City, Okla

John Astin, PhD
Complementary and Alternative
  Medicine Program
Stanford University
Palo Alto, Calif

Glenna Batson, PT, MA
Division of Occupational Therapy
University of North Carolina,
  Chapel Hill
Chapel Hill, NC

Forrest Batz, PharmD
PhytoMedicine Education
Santa Rosa, Calif

Mark Blumenthal
President
American Botanical Council
Austin, Texas

Deborah Bowes, PT, CFT
Feldenkrais Center for Movement
  Education
San Francisco, Calif

Dwight C. Byers
President
International Institute of Reflexology
St. Petersburg, Fla

John Cardellina II
Vice president
Council for Responsible Nutrition
Washington, DC

Jack F. Carter, PhD
President
Flax Institute of the United States
Fargo, ND

Theodore Cherbuliez, MD
President
American Apitherapy Society
Hillsboro, Calif

Peter Barry Chowka
Public and National Affairs Consultant
American Association of Naturo-
  pathic Physicians
Seattle, Wash

Carol M. Davis, EdD, PT
Associate Professor of Physical Therapy
University of Miami School of
  Medicine
Miami, Fla

James A. Duke, PhD
Botanical Consultant
Fulton, Md

Michael Reed Gach, PhD
Director
Acupressure Institute
Berkeley, Calif

Scott Gerson, MD
Medical Director
The National Institute of
  Ayurvedic Medicine
Brewster, NY

Hope Gillerman
NASTAT-Certified Alexander
  Technique Instructor
New York, NY

Elliot Greene, MA, NCTMB
Former President
American Massage Therapy Association
Silver Spring, Md

Curtiss D. Hunt, PhD
Research Biologist
USDA ARS Grand Forks Human
  Nutrition Research Center
Grand Forks, ND

Stanley W. Jacob, MD
Gerlinger Professor
Oregon Health Sciences University
Portland, Ore

Joanne M. Jordan, MD, MPH
Research Associate Professor
Thurston Arthritis Research Center
University of North Carolina School
  of Medicine
Chapel Hill, NC

Jon Kabat-Zinn, PhD
Executive Director
Center for Mindfulness in
  Medicine, Health Care and Society
University of Massachusetts
  Medical Center
Worchester, Mass

Joel Kremer, MD
Chief of Rheumatology
Albany Medical College
Albany, NY

Robert Lahita, MD
Chief of Rheumatology
St. Luke's Roosevelt Hospital
New York, NY

Judith Lasater, PhD, PT
Iyengar Yoga Instructor
San Francisco, Calif

Martin Lee, PhD
Founder
Tai Chi Cultural Center
Los Altos, Calif

Kate Lorig, DrPH, RN
Associate Professor of Medicine
Stanford University School of Medicine
Palo Alto, Calif

Dale A. Matthews, MD
Georgetown University School
  of Medicine
Washington, DC

Robert S. Maurer, DO
Executive Secretary
American Osteopathic College
  of Rheumatology
Edison, NJ

Jerome F. McAndrews, DC
National Spokesperson
American Chiropractic Association
Arlington, Va

David McCurdy, DMin
The Park Ridge Center for the Study
  of Health, Faith and Ethics
Chicago, Ill

James McKoy, MD
Chief of Rheumatology
Kaiser Permanente
Honolulu, Hawaii

Jeanne L. Melvin, MS, OTR
Chronic Pain and Fibromyalgia
  Management Program
Cedars-Sinai Medical Center
Los Angeles, Calif

Don Miller, PharmD, FASHP
Chair, Department of Pharmacy Practice
North Dakota State University
Fargo, ND

David Molony, LiscAc, Certified Chinese Herbalist (NCCAOM)
Executive Director
The American Association of Oriental Medicine
Catasauqua, Pa

Sarah Morgan, MD, MS, RD, FADA, FACP
Associate Professor of Nutrition Sciences and Medicine
University of Alabama at Birmingham
Birmingham, Ala

Charles Mraz
Beekeeper
Middlebury, Vt

Meena Narula, MS, PT
Feldenkrais Practitioner
Rochester, Minn

Michele Petri, MD
Director, The Lupus Center
Johns Hopkins University School of Medicine
Baltimore, Md

Martin Rossman, MD
Academy for Guided Imagery
Mill Valley, Calif

Ronenn Roubenoff, MD, MHS, FACP, FACR
Associate Professor of Medicine and Nutrition
Jean Mayer USDA Human Nutrition Research Center on Aging
Tufts University
Boston, Mass

Richard P. Sloan, PhD
Behavioral Medicine Program
Columbia-Presbyterian Medical Center
New York, NY

Touch Research Institute
University of Miami School of Medicine
Miami, Fla

David H. Trock, MD, FACP
Chief, Section of Rheumatology
Danbury Hospital
Danbury, Conn

Dana Ullman, MPH
President
Homeopathic Educational Services
Berkeley, Calif

Ferris Urbanowski, MA
Center for Mindfulness in Medicine, Health Care and Society
University of Massachusetts Medical Center
Worchester, Mass

Michael I. Weintraub, MD
New York Medical College
Valhalla, NY

Kathryn Williams, MD
Rehabilitation Specialist
Martinez, Calif

Jackie Wooton
Alternative Medicine Foundation, Inc.
Bethesda, Md

Yoga Research Center
Lower Lake, Calif

Robert B. Zurier, MD
Director, Rheumatology Division
University of Massachusetts Medical School
Worchester, Mass

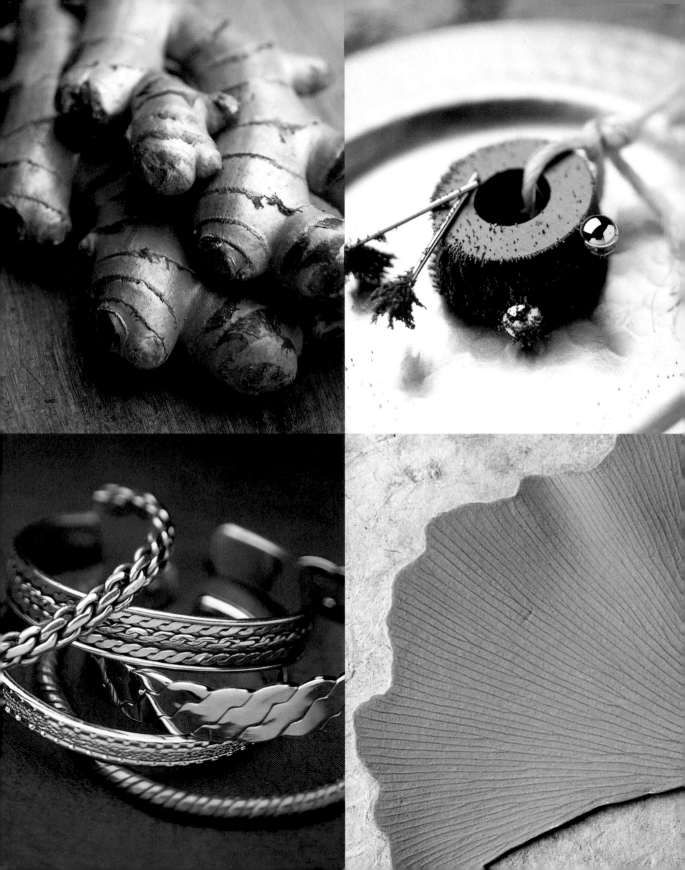

Introduction

Chronic disease can grind the joy and meaning right out of your life. Pain and disability isolate you from friends and activities you used to enjoy. Fatigue and stress make you vulnerable to other ailments. There is no cure for most kinds of arthritis, and the limited treatments available can leave you feeling helpless, frustrated and depressed. When it seems like you've come to the end of what conventional medicine has to offer and you're still sick and hurting, you may be willing to try anything.

It's no wonder, then, that so many of the 43 million people with arthritis are looking at alternative therapies. In fact, you may already be using some: According to a 1998 survey, nearly half of all Americans are trying some kind of unconventional therapy.

Some of these treatments and remedies can help you live a healthier life. They have thousands of years of tradition behind them, and scientific studies are showing they can be effective. Meditation is one good example: It's now an accepted treatment for stress, anxiety and pain. You may even find it – along with yoga and acupuncture – at your local hospital or health-care center, or offered through your health maintenance organization.

But quite a few of the more popular alternative therapies are useless, and some are dangerous. Hucksters abound, preying on your pain and promoting questionable treatments that promise "cures" for incurable diseases and "miracle" treatments that do everything but your dishes. Dietary supplements especially, with their promise of "natural" healing, vary greatly in effectiveness, quality and safety. These fake treatments can do more than take your money and raise false hopes. Even if they aren't outright dangerous, they may harm you by keeping you from using proven therapies.

This book is not about alternative "cures." It's intended as a common-sense guide through the maze of the most-used complementary therapies for arthritis, to help you choose wisely among the many options available.

Until well into the 20th century, many of the therapies we now call alternative were mainstream medicine: There *were* no alternatives. Surgery was risky, infections often fatal. Doctors prescribed herbs and other plant-based medicines, and did massage and manipulations. Mental attitudes, such as faith and the will to live, were considered an important part of healing, and prevention was a major form of health care. Many of these therapies are still considered mainstream medicine in other cultures.

What Complementary Medicine Might Do for You

What complementary medicine can do:

- Help you take an active role in your health care.
- Ease some symptoms, especially pain, stiffness, stress, anxiety and depression.
- Improve your outlook, your attitude and the quality of your life.
- Work with conventional medicine to enhance the effects of both kinds of treatments, and promote wellness.

What complementary medicine can't do:

- Treat most acute illnesses.
- Replace proven medical treatments.
- "Cure" chronic disease.

Meanwhile, advances in medical science led Western medicine to a more technical, intervention-based health care. The results have been spectacular. Vaccines protect us from a range of deadly diseases, antibiotics are truly lifesavers, and surgery can perform wonders. It has extended our life span from an average age of 48 at the turn of the 20th century to 76 as we enter the millennium. With these advances in medical technology, most medical schools stopped teaching older, time-consuming treatments.

Why, then, do so many people want to turn back the clock by returning to complementary medicine?

Part of it is frustration with today's impersonal health-care system. But much of the interest in alternatives is due to disappointment that so few of these dramatic medical successes have come for chronic illnesses such as arthritis. Although Western medicine excels at treating acute ills such as infections, emergencies and accidents, there are still relatively few treatments for illnesses that drag out over years or even decades. We are living longer with chronic diseases that are more complex to treat. They usually have more than one cause, and no simple solutions.

Alternative therapies may offer tools and remedies that, along with mainstream medicine, can influence your overall health. It's known that emotions and mental attitudes can have a major impact in the long-term management of chronic illness, for example. An interest in alternative therapies shows that you want

Defining the Terms

The phrase alternative and complementary medicine covers a broad range of healing philosophies, approaches and therapies. The National Institutes of Health says it generally is defined in the United States as those treatments and health-care practices that are not taught widely in medical schools, not generally used in hospitals, and not usually reimbursed by medical insurance companies. These therapies are also often called "unconventional therapies," since they are outside of mainstream Western medicine. Most often these therapies have not undergone rigorous scientific analysis.

Alternative medicine is a term that, until recently, was used for all unconventional therapies. It is still the term most commonly used today (hence the title of this book). However, it often refers to medical practices or remedies to be used *in place of* mainstream Western medicine, such as exclusive use of herbs, or of so-called "natural healing therapies" instead of prescription drugs. We at the Arthritis Foundation believe this approach is too narrow, because it doesn't take advantage of the proven benefits of conventional medicine.

Complementary medicine better describes the Arthritis Foundation's approach to unconventional therapies. Complementary therapies are used along with or in support of mainstream Western medicine. We will use the term complementary medicine throughout this book, because any treatments you try we would like you to use along with your conventional medical treatments.

Some other terms you may hear include:

Western medicine, allopathic medicine. These terms refer to the medical treatments and therapies – drugs and otherwise – accepted by U.S. mainstream medicine, taught in medical schools, and used in hospitals. Although we have included it as an alternative healing system in this book, osteopathic medicine has been accepted into mainstream medicine. We decided to include it anyway because it is not commonly known to the public.

Holistic medicine. This term generally refers to a philosophy of medicine in which the health-care practitioner considers the physical, mental, emotional and spiritual aspects of a person in planning treatments and promoting the healing process.

Integrative medicine. This recently introduced term reflects a shift in philosophy among some medical professionals. It describes medical care that integrates complementary therapies into Western medical practice to use what's most appropriate to treat the individual.

Preventive medicine. In this aspect of medical practice, the practitioner educates and treats the person to prevent health problems from arising, rather than treat symptoms after problems have occurred. Typically this at least includes counseling on healthy life habits, performing certain screening tests, and immunizing.

Unconventional medicine. This term is used for any treatment or therapy – drugs or otherwise – that does not fall within the realm of conventional or Western medicine.

To learn more about the various types of arthritis and other musculoskeletal disorders, and the conventional therapies used to treat them, see Appendix A, page 236.

to take a more active role in your health care, and the sense of control that you gain by becoming involved in managing your arthritis can contribute to your overall well-being.

Until recently, many doctors have been reluctant to consider unconventional therapies. Few of these therapies have been studied with scientific methods, and most lack solid evidence to show if they are safe or effective. Because most medical schools don't teach unconventional therapies, few doctors know which might be useful. This is beginning to change – due to people like you who are living longer with ailments that can't be fixed with conventional medicine. Your determination to find effective treatments has spurred serious scientific research into many complementary therapies. As studies are completed, more evidence will be available

to help you and your physician choose between the good, the bad and the useless.

In the meantime, what should you do?

Make informed decisions. Read this book with care, and show it to your doctor. It will tell you about the scientific evidence (or lack of it), whether experts think a therapy might be worth trying regardless of whether there is scientific proof, and what precautions to take.

Use common sense. There's no free lunch, and there are no miracle cures for arthritis. Unconventional therapies are remedies that, along with mainstream medicine, may improve your symptoms – and may not. Weigh the risks and benefits as well as the costs in time and money, and know when to quit a therapy that isn't working for you. Ask your doctor to be your partner as you explore adding unconventional therapies to your treatment plan.

Don't expect a "cure" from complementary therapies. We can't repeat this enough: There is no cure for most kinds of arthritis. But some of these therapies can help you gain control over your health care, and regain control over your life. When used in combination with conventional medicine, they may help you feel better and live a fuller life.

Therapies and Their Uses

Read individual entries to learn about the research behind the claims.

THERAPY	SYMPTOM					USES AND COMMENTS
	PAIN	STIFFNESS	FATIGUE	INFLAMMATION	ANXIETY/DEPRESSION	
MEDITATION	●				●	Used also for stress, IBS and skin problems (psoriasis)
BIOFEEDBACK	●	●	●			Used also for IBS, insomnia, Raynaud's, lupus and scleroderma
VISUALIZATION	●				●	Used also for IBS, immune function
HYPNOSIS	●				●	Used also for IBS
RELAXATION	●				●	Used also for IBS, Raynaud's, sleep problems
PRAYER	●				●	
YOGA	●	●	●		●	Improves energy, balance and function
TAI CHI	●	●	●		●	Improves energy, balance and function
QI GONG	●	●	●		●	Improves energy, balance and function
ALEXANDER	●	●				Improves balance and function
FELDENKRAIS	●	●				Improves balance and function
TRAGER	●	●				Improves balance and function
MASSAGE	●	●	●		●	Improves function; relieves stress; moderates immune system; used also for IBS
ACUPUNCTURE	●	●		●	●	Used also for nausea, fibromyalgia, Raynaud's, IBS
BEE VENOM	●	●		●		Used also for fibromyalgia
COPPER BRACELETS				●		
L.E.L.L.	●			●		Used for fibromyalgia, carpal tunnel
MAGNETS	●	●		●		
P.E.M.	●	●				Used for OA; not available in the U.S.
FASTING	●	●		●		
VEGETARIAN DIET	●	●		●		
HERBS AND SUPPLEMENTS						See page 188 for chart of herbs

PATIENT ADVICE

Before You Commit to a Complementary Therapy

If you're going to experiment with unproven therapies, be sure to protect yourself. Remember the basic principle of conventional treatment that all physicians observe: First, do no harm.

To minimize the chance that you might unintentionally harm yourself, here are some common-sense suggestions to consider before you decide to try a complementary therapy.

- Get an accurate diagnosis. Make sure you know from your physician specifically what

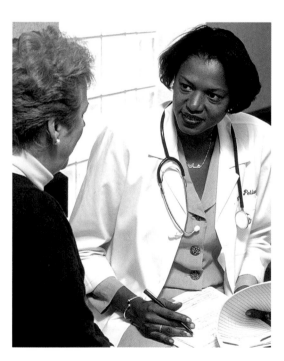

type of arthritis or musculoskeletal disorder you have, so you know what you're treating.

- Ask your doctor. Is this a therapy that might help my condition? Will there be any interaction between this therapy and the medications or other treatments you're giving me? (See Working with Your Doctor and Complementary Medicine, page 11).

- Get information. Check the Resources section for each therapy, and contact professional organizations to learn more about the therapy. Your local library is a good source (see Building Your Knowledge, page 16).

- Check references. Talk to others who have gone through the treatment – both those treated recently and those treated in the past. Ask their opinions about the advantages and disadvantages, risks, side effects, costs and their results.

- Check qualifications. If the therapy is regulated, does the practitioner have a license or certificate? Is he or she certified by a professional organization? Where did the practitioner get his or her training?

- Consider the cost. How much time and money do you have to invest? Ask how much it costs and how many treatments you'll need to see some effect. Complementary treatments are not usually covered by health insurance.

Tip-Offs to Rip-Offs

New health frauds pop up all the time, but the promoters usually fall back on the same old clichés and tricks to gain your trust and get your money. The National Center for Complementary and Alternative Medicine says the following are red flags for fraud:

- The vendor or practitioner claims the treatment or product works by a secret formula. Legitimate scientists share their knowledge so their peers can review the data.

- There are claims that the treatment is an amazing or miraculous breakthrough or a "cure." Real medical breakthroughs are few and far between, and when they happen, they're not touted as "amazing" or "miraculous" by any responsible scientist or journalist.

- The treatment is publicized only in the back pages of magazines, over the phone, by direct mail, in newspaper ads that pretend to be news stories, or on 30-minute commercials in talk show format ("infomercials"). The results of studies on bona fide treatments are generally reported first in medical journals.

- "Proof" for the treatment relies solely on testimonials from satisfied customers. These people may never have had the disease the product is supposed to cure, may be paid representatives, or may simply not exist. Often they're identified only by initials or first names.

Seven Danger Signs About A Therapist

Some types of complementary medicine are regulated and many practitioners have high standards of professional ethics and practice. However, others are not regulated – and unfortunately, not all practitioners are ethical or competent.

Be suspicious of any health professional who

- promises you can be "cured." Many therapies may help your condition, but there is no cure for most kinds of arthritis and related diseases – and no reputable practitioner will promise a cure.

- tells you to stop or decrease prescription medications. Never stop or change doses of prescription drugs without talking to your physician. Stopping certain medications (such as glucocorticoids like cortisone) abruptly can be dangerous. Other drugs may be necessary to keep your overall management program in balance. Stopping some prescription drugs, especially those for rheumatoid arthritis or lupus, can lead to flares of disease activity.

- advises a severely restricted diet. No, we don't mean a vegetarian diet – we mean a diet that is extreme or involves eliminating many types of foods. If you want to go this route, ask your doctor for a referral to a nutritionally oriented physician or to a registered dietitian with expertise in arthritis who will help you plan a well-balanced diet.
- insists you pay in advance for a series of expensive treatments. No practitioner can predict how you might respond to a treatment, and you should not have to pay for treatments you do not receive or need.

- cannot show you a license or a certificate from an approved school or organization in his or her specialty. Anyone can claim to be an "expert:" Ask for proof. (See information about certification in each therapy section.)
- advises you to keep the treatment a secret from your doctor, or anyone else. Good medical treatments are not secrets – they are shared in the medical community. Your doctor and your spouse or partner (or at least one member of your family or good friend) should know the details of your medical treatment, in case of emergency.
- suggests or asks for an intimate sexual relationship. This is totally inappropriate behavior. Any practitioner who crosses this boundary should be reported to the state medical board of registration, or the appropriate licensing or certifying agency for that therapy.

WORKING WITH YOUR DOCTOR AND COMPLEMENTARY MEDICINE

In ever increasing numbers, people want to take charge of their health. This is a smart move for those who have chronic ailments. To be successful, you need support and advice from a health professional.

Yet studies show that two-thirds of those using some form of complementary medicine don't tell their doctors. They give many reasons, but the major one is concern their doctor will disapprove or even stop treating them.

It's true that not all doctors approve of complementary therapies. However, it's in your best interest to keep your doctors informed. Every therapy that's strong enough to help you is also strong enough to hurt you. Your doctor can't give you the best possible professional advice without knowing all of the treatments you are using – whether they are over-the-counter drugs such as ibuprofen, or herbal remedies, nutritional supplements and exercise programs.

Here are some tips for helping you and your physician work together.

- Always tell you doctor everything you are taking or doing, including over-the-counter drugs, herbs, vitamins and special diets or exercises.
- Talk to your doctor before consulting a complementary medicine practitioner. Don't assume your doctor will be negative: Many doctors work with complementary medicine therapists and can steer you to a good practitioner.
- Ask what your doctor knows about this particular remedy – and listen carefully to what your doctor says.
- If your doctor is negative about this therapy, ask for a detailed explanation.
- If you doctor doesn't know about the therapy you wish to try, offer information. See the Resources section in each chapter for where to find more information, and check Appendix C to find studies from medical journals that you can show to your doctor.
- If your doctor approves or doesn't object, ask for a prescription or referral. The therapy may be covered by your health insurance if your doctor prescribes it.
- Expect the same cooperation from the complementary medicine therapist.

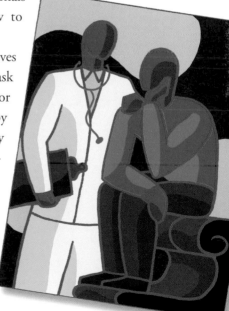

Getting the Most of Any Treatment

Here are some basic guidelines for getting good health care, no matter what kind of therapy you are using.

- Decide how much you want to know about and participate in your medical treatment, and tell your doctor your decision. If you don't want to be responsible for details of your health care, complementary therapies may not be a good option for you.

- Ask for regular evaluations of your long-term medication and treatment plan. Most doctors like to do this every year or so for patients with chronic ailments. This is a good time to discuss the benefits of your current treatment plan, and possible changes.

- Ask for enough time for a discussion. When you have something you want to talk about – such as a change in treatment or a complementary therapy you are considering – don't surprise your doctor. Ask in advance for an appointment that allows enough time for you to have a discussion.

- Be prepared. It's hard to remember everything you want to say, and everything a doctor tells you. Make a list of what you want to discuss and bring it to the appointment. Keep notes about what you discuss. You may want to bring a friend or a tape recorder to be sure you get the information right. Ask permission before you tape a consultation. Explain that you may not be able to remember everything and want to be able to replay it later.

- Keep your own medical records. Because you have a chronic ailment, you will see many different health-care professionals over time. Or you may move, or become ill while visiting far from home. It's important to have your medical records in one place; and it's especially important to keep records if you are using unconventional therapies.

- Keep a list with you of all medications *of all kinds* that you are taking. Be sure to include any reactions you've had or treatments that were not effective. Some people keep this information on an index card in their wallet. It can save time in an emergency, and is useful to take when you see new physicians or health practitioners.

If Your Doctor Refuses to Consider Complementary Medicine

It's difficult when the person you entrust with your health care won't talk about issues you consider important. You might want to ask for an office visit where you can discuss the kind of treatment each of you expects.

You have other options:

- Get a second opinion. You may have to pay for this yourself, but it is a possibility.
- Change doctors. This is a drastic step, especially if you have a long relationship with your doctor and have been satisfied with your overall medical treatment. You need to consider how important complementary care is to you.
- Above all, don't go behind your doctor's back by using therapies without telling him or her. All good relationships are based on trust and mutual respect. When you are not honest with your doctor, you are setting up a bad situation – and maybe even a medical emergency.

HOW TO USE THIS BOOK

This book is organized by types of therapy, with similar ones grouped together.

In each chapter, you'll find:

- a description of the therapy and how it is used
- scientific evidence about the therapy
- expert opinion of the therapy
- how to find a practitioner
- what the therapy costs
- resources on how and where to learn more.

To find out which might be useful for your condition, see the chart on page 7. It cross-references symptoms with therapies that may help relieve them.

Sources. Throughout the text, you'll see a name in parentheses just about every time a study is cited. That's the name of the lead researcher of the study. You can find the citation for these studies in the Appendix C section that matches the chapter.

Resources. This book can't report on all of the therapies available or tell everything about them, but it can tell you where to find out more. At the end of each therapy, there is a resource section listing organizations, books, video and audio tapes, and Web sites. There is also a section on Recommended Reading in Appendix B. For tips on how to use these resources, see Building Your Knowledge, page 16.

Looking at the Scientific Evidence

In researching this book, we searched medical journals, interviewed researchers and examined manufacturers' claims to bring you the soundest and most reliable information available to us. Quite often, there were no or few studies available for the therapies discussed here, and in most cases the studies that were available did not look at arthritis specifically. Also, many studies of complementary therapies are conducted in other countries. These reports are published in languages other than English, making some of them inaccessible to us.

Throughout this book, we've tried to indicate the quality of the studies we cited. Although we've tried to use straightforward language, it's nearly impossible to avoid using the language of science when talking about clinical and basic science research. So here's an explanation of the terms we'll be using in the rest of the book.

The term **study** is used very loosely to refer to any analysis. That can range from one researcher's observations of one patient (often called an **anecdote**) to a major undertaking involving hundreds of patients at many medical centers.

We've taken care to tell you whether the studies were done in test tubes, on animals or with humans. There's a big difference. A **test tube study** can identify the activities of some chemicals on cells, such as the anti-inflammatory properties of the herb ginger. However, just because a substance demonstrates certain properties in the test tube does not mean the substance will have an effect in a whole organism. **Animal studies** (usually on mice or rats) can show effects in living creatures. Animal and test tube studies are often called **preclinical trials.**

Although preclinical trials give useful information, such studies can't completely predict how a treatment will work on humans. Only with human studies can we know for sure how something will affect a person – and that it is safe. Studies on humans are called **clinical trials.**

A **controlled trial** compares the effects of a treatment on two or more groups of people. The **experimental** group gets the active treatment being studied. The **control** group may get a different treatment or an inactive treatment called a **placebo**. Sometimes, there are several groups of patients in a study who get different treatments. This way, researchers can compare the effects of the treatment being studied to several presently available therapies at once.

To make sure the outcome of the study isn't biased or influenced by pre-existing differences among patients assigned to the study groups, some trials are **randomized** (researchers assign people at random to either the experimental group or the placebo group). To make sure the power of suggestion does not affect the results, studies are **blinded:** In a **single-blind** study, the people being studied aren't told which treatment they are getting. In a **double-blind** study, both the patients and the researchers are "blind" to who is getting the tested substance or who is getting the placebo.

Most scientists consider the gold standard for clinical trials to be a **randomized, double-blind, placebo-controlled clinical trial.** For the results to be taken seriously, the improvement caused by the study treatment must be **statistically significant**, which means analysis must show the difference between the treatment and the placebo group was large enough so that it wasn't due to chance. As many as 30 percent of the people taking a placebo report positive effects, so if the treatment being studied does not have a better result than the placebo, it's not considered effective.

Other factors to consider when evaluating a study:

• Is the study published in a peer-reviewed medical journal, such as *The New England Journal of Medicine* or *Arthritis and Rheumatism*? To be in these journals, a study has to be examined by experts in the field who agree it meets accepted scientific standards. This eliminates many studies that aren't well done.

• How long was the therapy studied? A few weeks or months may show that something can have an effect, but doesn't show its long-term effects – or safety.

- Who performed the study, and where was it done? Good research can come from many sources. But trials performed by recognized experts at a major university or medical center tend to carry more weight.
- Who paid for the study? If the research was financed by a company who has a financial interest in the outcome, the results can very well be accurate – but there is always the possibility of conflict of interest and bias. Published studies will say how they were funded.
- Does the researcher have a financial interest in the therapy? In reputable, peer-reviewed journals, researchers must declare potential conflicts of interest, such as financial, that could influence their opinions or interpretation of the outcomes of the study.
- How many studies show the same result? One study may come to the wrong conclusion but when the results are confirmed over and over again, you can be re-assured the results are valid.

Building Your Knowledge

Knowledge is power, and with today's resources you can become your own expert on therapies that interest you. Here's some advice.

Organizations

Each therapy section has a list of organizations that represent it. Most will send you free information, or referrals to practitioners in your area. But remember: These organizations have a vested interest in the therapies and practitioners they represent, so use your judgment when looking at materials. Always seek confirmation of any claims from more than one source, including your doctor. Appendix E includes a list of organizations that represent several kinds of arthritis conditions. These are good sources to get a more conservative point of view about complementary therapies. Many organizations have a toll-free hotline for questions, and an Internet site.

Libraries

Your public library can be an excellent source of information. And it's free. There you will find books, video and audio tapes, and also access to data bases (articles stored on CD-ROMs or computers) and to the Internet. Almost all information these days is online and available through a computer – even the library file catalogue. Libraries have instructions on how to use their systems as well as how to access the Internet. If you aren't experienced in using computers, don't worry. Ask a librarian for help. If you don't wish to talk about your own situation, say that you're gathering background material for an article you are writing.

A library is also a place to sample before you buy expensive books. Research moves quickly these days: Many books more than three years old may no longer be accurate. And check the source. There's lots of misinformation out there. Articles in magazines and newspapers and even books may emphasize the dramatic, or have a point of view to sell you. Depend on established, respected sources such as medical journals and books by respected experts. When in doubt, ask your health-care professionals.

Your local reference librarian can help you find sources of information, and order books or other materials through interlibrary loan. Medical journals are not usually found in public libraries, but today's computer technology puts the National Library of Medicine as close as your public library – closer, if you have a computer and a modem at home.

Using the Internet

The most up-to-date information today is found on the Internet in Web sites. You don't have to own a computer, or know anything about computers: Most public libraries have free access, and a librarian can show you how to use the Internet. You can go to the home pages of the National Center for Complementary and Alternative Medicine, and to many medical organizations.

But surf with care: Web sites abound, because anyone can put a site up on the Internet, and not all of them offer accurate or timely information. The Net is also loaded with opportunists who want to sell you something.

You can look for articles cited in this book on the Internet for free by contacting MEDLINE, a service of The National Library of Medicine at http://igm.nlm.nih.gov. It has millions of articles on file. You will find abstracts (summaries of articles) online, but not the whole article. If you want the whole article, you can contact the journal and order a reprint. The price of a reprint varies.

The National Center for Complementary and Alternative Medicine also has a Web site with much good information at http://nccam.nih.gov.

We've listed trustworthy Web sites in each section, and in Appendix B. (See Useful Web Sites, page 251). At the time of publication, the Web sites listed in this book were reliable and up-to-date, but Web site contents and even addresses change frequently. You'll find that many of them are linked to each other, or to other sites, and that some information is duplicated on many sites.

If You Can't Do Your Own Searching

If you can't do your own searching, you can pay a professional researcher to find answers to your health questions.

MedCetera Inc., in Houston, Texas, offers several packages ranging from a basic MEDLINE printout to more extensive searches that can supply full-text articles. A basic MEDLINE search that doesn't include full-text articles at MedCetera costs $89 plus shipping. Phone: 800/748-6866.

The Health Resource Inc., in Conway, Ark, provides comprehensive search reports on specific medical conditions. Health Resource Inc.'s reports start at $195. Phone: 800/949-0090.

The Institute for Health and Healing Library (The Planetree Health Resource Center) at the California Pacific Medical Center in San Francisco is a nonprofit health and medical library open to the public that will also do searches. Fees range from about $50 for a basic search to $125 for an in-depth packet. Phone: 415/923-3681. E-mail: dakini@clas.org

The World Research Foundation in Sedona, Ariz, a nonprofit service, will provide search reports on complementary therapies from a mixture of sources that range from ancient texts to the current published studies. An average packet of 500 pages costs about $60. Phone: 520/284-3300. Web site: http://www.wrf.org.

Finding a Complementary Medicine Practitioner

In each section, you'll find organizations that represent each therapy and information on how to find a practitioner of that therapy. The resources below are more general, and include referrals to medical doctors, osteopaths and other licensed health professionals who practice holistic medicine and offer complementary therapies.

American Holistic Health Association
P.O. Box 17400
Anaheim, CA 92817-7400
Phone: 714/779-6152
E-mail: ahha@healthy.net
Web site: http://ahha.org
Offers a list of licensed or certified practitioners who have an active practice and holistic approach in a recognized field of wellness or health care.

American Holistic Medical Association
6728 Old McLean Village Drive
McLean, VA 22101
Phone: 703/556-9327
Web site: http://www.holisticmedicine.org
An association of MDs, DOs and other licensed health-care practitioners with a holistic approach to health care. Members are listed on the Web site, or a full directory is available by mail for $10.

A Glossary of Health-Professional Titles

It can be daunting to try to figure out those initials after a health professional's name. The list below explains some of the titles you may see; it does not include every medical title. We've given a bit of an explanation for the less-common ones.

AAMA: The practitioner is a member of the American Academy of Medical Acupuncturists, which is open only to medical doctors (MD) and doctors of osteopathy (DO).

ATI, MATI: Designates teaching members of Alexander Technique International (the "M" is optional).

BAMS: Bachelor of Ayurvedic Medicine. The practitioner has completed an approved program at an ayurvedic university in India or Sri Lanka.

BCIAC: Refers to Biofeedback Certification Institute of America certification.

BSW, MSW: Bachelor of science in social work, master's of science in social work. Social workers offer a broad range of services from emotional support to referrals for community resources. Most states require social workers to pass a licensing exam.

CA: Certified Acupuncturist. Certified by state-approved program.

CAR: Certified Advanced Rolfer. Designates a Certified Rolfer (CR) with at least three years' certification and continuing education credits who has completed additional course work from the Rolf Institute.

CCH: Certified to practice classical homeopathy; available to all professionals through the Council for Homeopathic Certification.

CR: Certified Rolfer. This designation requires training at the Rolf Institute and a college-level understanding of anatomy, physiology, kinesiology and psychology.

DAc: May indicate advanced training in acupuncture. Also used as a licensure title in some states instead of Licensed Acupuncturist.

DAMS: Doctor of Ayurvedic Medicine and Surgery. The practitioner has completed an approved program at an ayurvedic university in India or Sri Lanka.

DC: Doctor of Chiropractic. Chiropractors are trained in four-year chiropractic colleges and are licensed in all 50 states. However, chiropractors are not medical doctors and are not licensed to perform surgery or prescribe drugs.

DHANP: Homeopathy certification available only to naturopathic practitioners through the Homeopathic Academy of Naturopathic Physicians.

DHt: Homeopathy certification available only to MDs and DOs through the American Board of Homeotherapeutics.

Dipl Ac: Diplomate in Acupuncture by the National Certification Commission for Acupuncture and Oriental Medicine.

DO: Doctor of Osteopathy. DOs complete a training, certification and licensing program that is almost exactly the same as that of an allopathic medical doctor (MD). They are licensed to perform surgery and write prescriptions.

DOM: Doctor of Oriental Medicine.

GCFP: Designates a guild-certified Feldenkrais practitioner, which requires completion of a professional training program accredited by the Feldenkrais Guild, including 800–1000 hours of training over a three- to four-year period.

LAc, LicAc: Licensed Acupuncturist.

LNC: Licensed nutritionist counselor.

MAc: Master of Acupuncture. Graduate of a masters level program in acupuncture accredited by the Accreditation Commission for Acupuncture and Oriental Medicine, which is recognized by the U.S. Department of Education.

MD: Doctor of Medicine.

MOM: Graduate of a masters program in Oriental medicine accredited by the Accreditation Commission for Acupuncture and Oriental Medicine.

NASTAT: Designates membership in the North American Society of Teachers of the Alexander Technique, which requires members to complete 1,600 hours of training over at least a three-year period at a NASTAT-certified school.

ND: Doctor of naturopathy. Naturopathic physicians undergo a four-year training program that includes training in homeopathy, clinical nutrition, manipulation, herbal medicine and hydrotherapy. It's best to consult one who is a graduate of one of the accredited naturopathic medical schools, and licensed.

NMD: Doctor of Naturopathic Medicine in the state of Arizona.

OMD or DOM: Designates an Oriental Medical Doctor or Doctor of Oriental Medicine, and refers to training beyond that required for a state acupuncture license. Chinese MDs who are licensed in China and U.S. practitioners who complete OMD or DOM degree programs at foreign schools also use these titles.

OT: Occupational Therapist.

PA: Physician Assistant.

PharmD: Doctor of Pharmacy.

PT: Physical Therapist.

RAc: Registered Acupuncturist. Licensure title used in some states for professional acupuncturists instead of Lac.

RN: Registered Nurse.

FOR MEDICAL PROFESSIONALS:
ABOUT THIS BOOK

Alternative medicine is everywhere: On the covers of major magazines, on prime-time TV, on the shelves of your local grocery store – perhaps even in your office reception room. And it's not going to go away. According to a 1998 Harvard University study, it's likely that nearly half of your patients are using some kind of alternative therapy, be it supplements, meditation, magnets, homeopathy or something more exotic. And two-thirds of them are not telling you about it (Eisenberg).

Those who live with chronic illness or pain, such as arthritis patients, are among the most likely to look beyond conventional medicine. They want your advice and support, but many are afraid to ask their physicians about alternatives or to admit they are using them for fear of your disapproval. They are also aware that most physicians simply don't know enough about these practices to be able to advise them.

This will change soon. Studies of alternative therapies are appearing in increasing numbers in medical journals, such as *Arthritis and Rheumatism*, and there are now several peer-reviewed journals devoted to alternative medicine (see page 23). The National Center for Complementary and Alternative Medicine is funding $50 million of research per year. Most medical schools have added at least one class in complementary medicine, and some are developing integrative medical programs such as the ones pioneered at the University of Maryland and the University of Arizona.

Our intent for this book is to give a balanced review of some of the most popular patient choices in complementary therapies for arthritis. We've laid out the available scientific evidence – or lack of it – along with some medical opinions and cautions. The quality and amount of research on complementary therapies varies widely. For some, there is no acceptable scientific evidence. Other therapies are well documented. We've indicated this in the text, and provided citations in the appendices for the studies mentioned. Along with reviews by the four physician editors, individual sections in the book have been reviewed by experts. You will find these expert reviewers' names and affiliations listed in the Acknowledgments section.

You may already be using one or more of the therapies in this book for yourself, your patients or both. You may not approve of others. Whatever your beliefs, it's important for you to know what your patients are doing. We urge you to talk with your patients about the remedies they are using, and to keep an open mind. Your patients with arthritis need your help and partnership in gaining control of their pain and regaining control of their lives.

The resources below are of special interest to health professionals. See also the many resources in each chapter and in the appendices.

Articles

Eisenberg DM, Davis RB, Ettner SL, Appel S, Wilkey S, VanRampay M, Kessler RC. Trends in alternative medicine use in the United States, 1990–1997. JAMA 1998; 280:1569–75.

Gordon NP, Sobel DS, Tarazona DS, Tarazona EZ. Use of and interest in alternative therapies among adult primary care clinicians and adult members in a large health maintenance organization. West J Med 1998; 169:153–61.

Journals

Alternative Therapies in Health and Medicine
This peer-reviewed journal focuses on the practical use of alternative therapies in the prevention and treatment of disease and in promoting health, and encourages the integration of alternative therapies with conventional medical practices.
Executive Editor: Larry Dossey, MD
Bimonthly. $6.95 per issue.
Web site: http://www.alternative-therapies.com

Complementary Therapies in Medicine
A peer-reviewed journal primarily for those whose background is in traditional health practices, and who are seeking objective and critical guidance and information about complementary therapies.
Editor-in-Chief: Andrew Vickers, Research Council for Complementary Medicine, London, United Kingdom
United States Editor: B. M. Berman, MD, University of Maryland, Baltimore
Published quarterly. $96.
Web site: http://www.churchillmed.com/Journals/CTMedicine/jhome.html

Integrative Medicine: Integrating Conventional and Alternative Medicine
A peer-reviewed journal that promotes health and healing by integrating concepts and techniques of allopathic, alternative and complementary medicine. Publishes original studies, critical review articles, major scientific reports, and insightful debates, providing balanced perspectives on health-care practices.
Editor-in-Chief: Andrew T. Weil, MD, University of Arizona College of Medicine, Tuscon
Published quarterly. $52.
Web site: http://www.elsevier.nl/inca/publications/store/6/0/0/7/5/9/

The International Journal of Integrative Medicine
Peer-reviewed journal presents information from mainstream and natural medicine perspectives.
Editor-in-Chief: Frances E. Fitzgerald
Bimonthly. $68 per year.
Web site: http://impakt.com

The Journal of Alternative and Complementary Medicine: Research on Paradigm, Practice and Policy
This peer-reviewed journal includes observational and analytical reports on treatments outside the realm of allopathic medicine. It includes current concepts in clinical care, including case reports that will be valuable for health-care professionals and scientists who are seeking to evaluate and integrate these therapies into patient care protocols and research strategies.
Editor-in-Chief: Kim A. Jobst, DM, MRCP, Glasgow Homeopathic Hospital and University, Glasgow, Scotland, United Kingdom
Published quarterly. $69 plus $12 (shipping & handling).
Web site: http://www.liebertpub.com/acm

Books
Alternative Medicine: Expanding Medical Horizons. By BM Berman, DB Larson and JP Swyers. NIH publication. Washington: U.S. Government Printing Office, 1992. $26.

Complementary Therapies in Rehabilitation: Holistic Approaches for Prevention and Wellness. Edited by Carol M. Davis. Thorofare, New Jersey: SLACK, 1997. Paperback. $35.

Fundamentals of Complementary and Alternative Medicine. Edited by Marc S. Micozzi. New York: Churchill Livingston, 1996. Paperback, with CD ROM. $46.

The Professional's Handbook of Complementary & Alternative Medicines. By Charles W. Fetrow and Juan R. Avila. Springhouse, PA: Springhouse Publishing, 1999. Paperback. $40.

Web Site and Clearinghouse
The National Center for Complementary and Alternative Medicine maintains a Web site and phone number for consumer information. This arm of the National Institutes of Health conducts and supports basic and applied research and training and disseminates information on complementary and alternative medicine to practitioners and the public. The Clearinghouse toll-free line focuses on NCCAM-funded research but will help with other sources for information on alternative therapies.
NCCAM Clearinghouse
PO Box 8218
Silver Spring, MD 20907-8218
Phone: 888/644-6226.
Web site: http://nccam.nih.gov

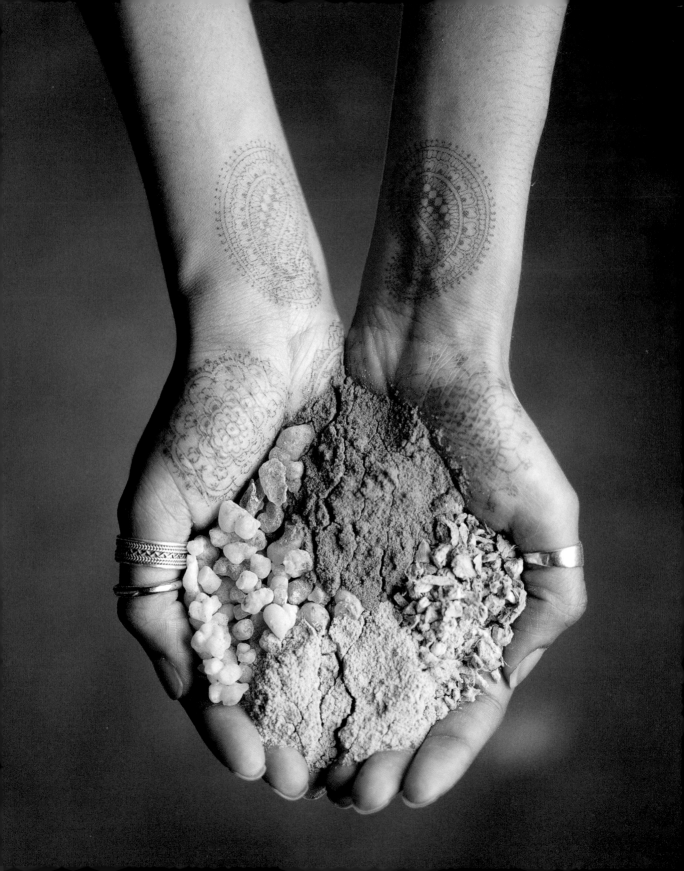

Alternative Healing Systems

OTHER APPROACHES TO
HEALTH AND HEALING

When most of us think of medical care, we think of mainstream Western-style medicine. That's one of the reasons therapies outside that tradition are called "alternative."

But for much of the world, our U.S. medicine is the "alternative": The National Center for Complementary and Alternative Medicine estimates that only 10 to 30 percent of human health care is delivered by conventional, biomedically oriented practitioners. The rest of the world receives health care that ranges from self-care and folk remedies to care given in an organized system based on an alternative tradition or practice.

Each major organized healing system (including allopathic medicine) has its own theory of health and disease; an educational program or organization to teach its concepts and certify its practitioners; and a system to maintain and regulate its practice.

Healing systems such as Chinese medicine and Indian ayurvedic medicine are mainstream medicine for billions of people. They have concepts of disease, health and healing that have little in common with our Western model, and practices and remedies that may be very different. Other healing systems, such as osteopathy and chiropractic, are very similar to Western medicine but have distinctly different underlying philosophies.

Many healing traditions were developed long before drugs and surgery were dependable and safe treatments. Thus the practices and treatments in many are aimed at discovering and restoring balance in the body through diet, exercise, mental attitude and the cultivation of vital life energy. Instead of seeing healing as a battle against disease, many traditions work from the premise that the body can heal itself and stay healthy with gentle remedies, many of them hands-on. These therapies often work very well along with Western medicine.

This section briefly reviews some of the best known alternative healing systems, and describes how each relates to Western medicine, and how it might help with your arthritis symptoms.

AYURVEDA: THE WISDOM OF THE BODY

Ayurveda, the ancient healing tradition of India, is perhaps the oldest of all medical systems. It originated more than 5,000 years ago in the Vedas, sacred Hindu texts that describe life in philosophical, spiritual and scientific terms. It's a comprehensive system that includes mental and spiritual well-being as well as physical health. The original goal of ayurveda, which means "science of life," was to maintain physical health and well-being so one could better pursue spiritual development.

Today, ayurveda remains a major form of health care in India, where it is often used along with modern Western medicine. It is less well known in the United States: There are probably fewer qualified ayurvedic practitioners in the United States than in any other alternative healing practice. Ayurveda has become better known since the 1960s when the Maharishi Mahesh Yogi brought transcendental meditation to the West; and since it was popularized by Deepak Chopra, MD, a Western-trained endocrinologist and prolific writer.

Key Principles and Practices

Ayurveda's key principles are based on vital life energy and spiritual, mental and physical balance. Its practices are noninvasive, focused on wellness and healthy living through diet, exercise, moderation and meditation. The practitioner is an advisor who suggests lifestyle and health practices to restore or optimize your mental, physical and spiritual well-being. It's up to you to put these practices to use. The success of ayurvedic therapy depends on your willingness to commit to a pattern of healthy daily living.

In ayurveda, all existence is made up of a vital life energy called prana, and of five key elements: earth, fire, water, air and ether. In humans, these elements are organized and expressed as three distinct types of physiological energies, called doshas. You may have heard doshas described, incorrectly, as "body types": doshas are body-soul-energy categories. The balance of the five elements is constantly shifting within doshas, in ourselves as well as in nature. Health is based on achieving harmony among these forces. Practices that help maintain and restore balance are yoga (see page 100), meditation (see page 62), vegetarian diet (see page 168), massage (see page 117) and purification regimens. The invisible and powerful life force of prana can be taken into the body through breath and enhanced through breathing exercises called pranayama.

What Happens in an Ayurvedic Treatment

Ayurvedic treatments are customized to each individual and his or her symptoms. The first session will last an hour or more. Follow-up visits are shorter and spaced weeks or months apart. The practitioner will take your pulse in several places, examine your tongue, and ask many questions about your diet, sleep and elimination habits, lifestyle preferences, and other characteristics to determine your predominant dosha. Then you will be given very specific diet advice, based on a vegetarian diet and tailored to your dosha and health situation. A daily routine of herbs, supplements and exercises will also be prescribed. It may include yoga postures (asanas) to simulate certain organs or muscles, and breathing exercises (pranayama) to balance your nervous system and enhance energy. Meditation is recommended to quiet the mind and allow "the wisdom of the body" to be heard.

Herbs and remedies are almost always given in combinations, either as formulations or prepared specifically for an individual and his or her symptoms. Many of these herbs are not found outside of India, and their names may be in Sanskrit. (See Ayurvedic Remedies, page 192.)

Digestion and elimination are very important in ayurveda, because it's believed a backup of toxins causes disease. For rheumatoid arthritis, fibromyalgia and many other chronic conditions, a series of purification treatments called panchakarma may be recommended to remove toxins and rebalance the body. These involve fasting, sweat baths and a routine to "clean out" the digestive system that can include vomiting, laxatives, enemas and other purging treatments. These cleansing sessions are given over several days at special centers, combined with deep rest and restorative massages.

What Ayurveda Offers People with Arthritis

Ayurveda sounds exotic, but its wellness-based practices work well with conventional medicine. In fact, many of its principles have probably already been recommended to you by your Western-trained doctor: Eat a balanced diet low in fats and rich in fresh fruits and vegetables; set up a daily routine that includes exercise and regular sleep; and reduce stress.

Studies have shown that many with chronic illness benefit from ayurvedic practices such as yoga, meditation and breathing exercises. (See Scientific Evidence sections for yoga, page 101; meditation, page 64; and relaxation techniques, page 81.)

There is evidence that some ayurvedic herbs help arthritis as well. (See Ayurvedic Remedies, page 192.)

There are few risks with ayurvedic medicine because its practices are noninvasive. However, herbs and remedies should be used with caution because they are not regulated as medications, and because some traditional remedies contain heavy metals. Look for a

RESORCES * AYURVEDA

Organizations

The organizations listed here offer training in ayurvedic medicine, and can give referrals to practitioners.

The Maharishi College of Vedic Medicine
2721 Arizona Street NE
Albuquerque, NM 87110
Phone: 505/830-0435 for consultations
Phone: 888/895-2614 for referral to a practitioner
E-mail: mcvmnm@aol.com
This organization was started by the same group that brought transcendental meditation to the West. It also markets a line of ayurvedic products. A related **Web site:** http://www.maharishi-medical.com

The National Institute of Ayurvedic Medicine
584 Milltown Road
Brewster, NY 10509
Phone: 888/246-NIAM (6426)
E-mail: niam@niam.com
Web site: http://www.niam.com

The Ayurvedic Institute
11311 Menaul NE
Albuquerque, NM 87112
Phone: 505/291-9698
Web site: http://www.ayurveda.com

The American School of Ayurvedic Sciences
2115 112th Avenue NE
Bellevue, WA 98004
Phone: 425/453-8022 for a referral to a practitioner

Books

Contemporary Ayurveda: Medicine and Research in Maharishi Ayur-Veda (Medical Guides to Complementary and Alternative Medicine), by Christopher Clark, Hari M. Sharma. 1997. Churchill Livingston. Paperback. $31.

Ayurveda : The Science of Self-Healing: A Practical Guide, by Vasant D. Lad. 1984. Lotus Light Publications. Paperback. $10.95.

Ayurveda: The Ancient Indian Healing Art, by Scott Gerson, MD. 1997. Element. Paperback. $9.95.

Ayurvedic Healing, by David Frawley. 1991. Morson Publishing. Paperback. $18.95.

Web Site

The Ayurveda Holistic Center
Has basic information and links to other ayurveda sites.
http://ayurvedahc.com/index.htm

---

practitioner experienced in ayurvedic remedies. Purification treatments involve some risks, so ask your doctor before undergoing intensive internal cleansing therapies.

Finding a Practitioner

There are not very many qualified ayurvedic practitioners in the United States. There is no U.S. national standard for certifying ayurvedic practitioners, so there is a wide range of expertise among those offering ayurveda. You need to choose a practitioner carefully. Graduates of Indian ayurvedic medical programs will have extensive knowledge. They will have a degree of BAMS (Bachelor of Ayurvedic Medicine and Surgery) or DAMS (Doctor of ayurvedic Medicine and Surgery) and will have completed a program at a qualified ayurvedic university in Asia. Others may have a strong subspecialty in ayurveda, or they may have just taken some courses and have little knowledge.

Experts recommend consulting a practitioner who has specialized in ayurvedic medicine and who has many years of experience. The ideal practitioner would be one who is trained in both ayurvedic and Western medicine such as a physician. You are also more likely to have your treatments covered by insurance if your receive them from a Western-trained physician, but it will be hard to find one.

To find a practitioner in your area, check the organizations listed in Resources. Those offering ayurvedic training may be able to refer you to practitioners.

Cautions

! Be careful taking ayurvedic herbal medicines with other drugs or herbs. Ask both the ayurvedic practitioner and your physician about possible interactions and side effects. Some herbs intensify the effects of drugs or other herbs.

! Purification treatments that involve equipment that enters your body may carry infection and have other risks. Be sure the facility and equipment are scrupulously clean. Consult with your doctor before undergoing internal cleansing treatments.

Costs

Fees vary widely. The first session may cost between $50 and $100, or more, depending on the credentials of the practitioner. Fees for follow-up visits are less. Panchakarma (intensive cleansing therapy) is done at a special facility; costs may range from $875-$2,500 for a four-day treatment. Yoga sessions generally cost $4-$20, and meditation instruction is taught free or for a flat fee that ranges from $40 to $600.

Health insurance generally doesn't pay for ayurvedic practices unless offered by a practitioner who is covered, such as a medical doctor.

CHINESE MEDICINE:
BALANCING VITAL ENERGY

Chinese medicine is perhaps the second oldest healing system, originating some 2,000 years ago. Many of the principles practiced today can be traced back to the Han Dynasty and a scholarly work called The Yellow Emperor's Book of Medicine.

Chinese medicine is widely used in Asia today, often along with allopathic medicine. Since the 1970s, it has become increasingly well known in the United States, especially for acupuncture and herbal medicine. Millions of people in the United States try acupuncture every year, primarily for pain. Many also practice tai chi chuan and qi gong, forms of exercise and moving meditation.

Key Principles and Practices

Chinese medicine evolved from observations of nature. Balance is at the heart of its principles and practices. This is expressed in the concepts of yin and yang and a vital life energy force called qi (pronounced chee). Yin and yang, which are sometimes called the feminine and masculine principles, represent the dynamic, inter-dependent but often opposing forces of nature.

Everyone – and everything – is a unique combination of yin and yang energies. Yin qualities are feminine, cool, passive and dark.

Yang energies are masculine, warm, active and bright. These two principles need to be balanced for optimal health, so every aspect of Chinese medicine involves the interaction of yin and yang.

Qi really has no English translation. Although commonly called vital life energy, it means much more than that. It is life itself, an invisible force that is in everything alive. In humans, qi flows through the body in invisible channels called meridians (which have no counterpart in the Western understanding of anatomy). When the flow of qi is blocked or out of balance, illness results.

Illness is described in terms of nature and qi qualities, and treatments are aimed at helping the person regain balance by unblocking – or strengthening – the flow of qi and the balance of yin and yang. The practices used for this include acupuncture (see page 135), acupressure, (see page 135), and exercises called tai chi chuan and qi gong (see page 107). In acupuncture, hair-fine needles are inserted at specific points along the meridians to stimulate the flow of qi. Acupressure, as the name implies, uses pressure rather than needles at acupoints. The ancient, dance-like movements of tai chi and qi gong are aimed at balancing qi as much as exercising the body.

Organizations
The American Association of Oriental Medicine
433 Front Street
Catasaugua, PA 18032
Phone: 888/500-7999 or 610/266-1433
Web site: http://www.aaom.org
Has a national referral list for Oriental medicine practitioners who are board-certified.

National Certification Commission for Acupuncture and Oriental Medicine
11 Canal Center Plaza, Suite 300
Alexandria, VA 22314
Phone: 703/548-9004
Web site: http://www.nccaom.org
Will send a list of traditional oriental medicine practitioners.

American Academy of Medical Acupuncture
5820 Wilshire Boulevard, Suite 500
Los Angeles, CA 90036
Phone: 323/937-5514
Web site: http://www.medicalacupuncture.org
Refers you to medical and osteopathic doctors who also practice acupuncture.

Books
The Web That Has No Weaver: Understanding Chinese Medicine, by Ted J. Kaptchuk. 1983. Lincolnwood, IL. NTC Publishing Group. Paperback. $18.95.

Between Heaven and Earth: A Guide to Chinese Medicine, by Harriet Beinfield and Efrem Korngold. 1992. New York. Ballantine Books. Paperback. $14.

The American Association of Oriental Medicine's Complete Guide to Chinese Herbal Medicine, by David Molony. 1998. New York. Berkeley Publishing Group. Paperback. $13.

Arthritis: The Chinese Way of Healing and Prevention, by Dr. Jwing-Ming Yang. 1996. Jamaica Plain, MA. YMAA Publication Center, Inc. Paperback. $16.95. Also on audio tape. $15.95.

Web Site
http://www.acupuncture.com

Herbal medicine plays a key role as well. Some individual Chinese herbs are well-known for certain properties (such as ginseng for stamina), but Chinese medicine practitioners usually prescribe herbs in combinations, custom-blended for a specific person and his or her specific situations (see Chinese herbs, page 198).

What Happens in a Chinese Medicine Treatment

In Chinese medicine, the practitioner looks for a pattern of symptoms or responses rather than a disease. The first session usually lasts an hour or more. Follow-up sessions are a week or months apart, and are usually much shorter. The practitioner will take your pulse in several places, examine your tongue, and ask many questions about your diet, sleep and elimination habits, lifestyle preferences, and other characteristics. The diagnosis terms don't relate to Western medicine: They will be described in terms of "qi deficiency" or "stagnation," or perhaps as cold, heat, wind, or damp of certain organs.

Treatment is customized to each individual. Most Americans who use Chinese medicine come for acupuncture. These sessions take from 20 minutes to an hour, and may be repeated every week or so until the condition improves. Some people return once or twice a year, usually in spring and fall, for a "tune-up." You may also be given diet advice and herbs.

What Chinese Medicine Offers People with Arthritis

Chinese medicine, with its emphasis on balance and healthy living, is well-suited to treating chronic illnesses. Acupuncture has been used successfully to ease the pain of many kinds of arthritis: Studies are mixed, but show best results for osteoarthritis and fibromyalgia. The gentle exercise of tai chi is a favorite for many who find movement painful; it's been shown to improve balance in the elderly. Qi gong may relieve stress and increase energy, and can be practiced with minimal movement. See Scientific Evidence for acupuncture, page 140; tai chi, page 109; and qi gong, page 109.

Herbs may also help many conditions connected with arthritis. A 1998 randomized, placebo-controlled trial of patients with irritable bowel syndrome found that those who received either a standardized Chinese herb formulation or a formula custom-designed for them both had significant improvements in symptoms compared to the placebo group (Bensoussan). See Chinese herbs, page 198.

There are few risks connected with Chinese medicine when provided by licensed or certified practitioners. In acupuncture, it's important to follow proper sterile procedures to prevent infections. Disposable needles are routinely used. Herbs should be used with caution because they are not regulated as medicines, and some herbs from Asia have been contaminated with heavy metals or pollutants. Look for an experienced and certified practitioner.

Finding a Practitioner

There are many people offering Chinese medicine in the United States. Because it is not a licensed medical practice in the United States, you may find a wide range of people dispensing herbs and claiming to be qualified practitioners.

At the time of publication, 38 states licensed acupuncturists. If your state doesn't require licensing, ask if the practitioner is certified by the National Certification Commission for Acupuncture and Oriental Medicine (NCCAOM): This national agency certifies acupuncturists and Chinese herbalists.

Contact the NCCAOM or one of the national certifying boards or agencies for a directory of practitioners. Medical doctors, naturopaths, chiropractors and many other health professionals offer acupuncture, all with different levels of expertise.

Look for someone who is certified and who has many years of experience.

Cautions

! Be careful taking Chinese herbal medicines with other drugs or herbs: Ask about possible interactions and side effects. Some herbs intensify the effects of drugs or other herbs.

! Almost all acupuncturists use disposable needles; nonetheless, ask to make sure.

Costs

Costs vary by location. A first acupuncture or acupressure visit may cost between $75 and $150. Follow-up visits cost between $35 and $75. These fees may include herbs. Some health insurers will cover these treatments, especially if prescribed by – or performed by – a physician.

NATUROPATHIC MEDICINE:
THE HEALING POWER OF NATURE

Naturopathic medicine evolved from the "natural cures" practiced in European spas in the 19th century. It was introduced to the United States by Bernard Lust who founded the American School of Naturopathy in 1896. It flourished throughout the United States, drawing thousands of patients. John Kellogg (of the breakfast cereals) used it in his health sanatorium in Battle Creek, Mich, and there were thousands of naturopathic physicians until the rise of pharmaceutical and high-tech treatments after World War II.

Naturopathy faded away for a few decades. Today, it's making a comeback. There are about 1,000 practitioners in the United States serving as primary care doctors who use therapies that are almost exclusively natural (hence the name naturopathic) and nontoxic.

Key Principles and Practices

The underlying principles of naturopathy revolve around encouraging healthy living habits and allowing the body to heal itself. The focus is on the person not the disease, and on working with the patient to prevent disease. Naturopathic medicine looks for disease causes in the patient's lifestyle, and uses the most gentle treatment possible. The doctor–patient relationship is cooperative, with the doctor acting as a teacher.

Health is achieved by removing poisons and bad habits, and encouraging exercise, good attitudes, and a balanced and moderate lifestyle. An eclectic mixture of treatments may include herbs and dietary supplements; nutrition; homeopathy; spinal manipulation; hydrotherapy; and counseling. Naturopathic practitioners are particularly known for their expertise in nutrition.

Modern naturopathic physicians (NDs) undergo a four-year training program that includes homeopathy, clinical nutrition, manipulation, herbal medicine and hydrotherapy. Many NDs have additional training and certification in Chinese medicine (both acupuncture and herbs), ayurveda and home birthing. They can treat wounds and are trained in minor surgery, but usually refer such treatments to physicians. They are not licensed to perform major surgery or to prescribe drugs. (In some states, they may prescribe certain medications, primarily those that come from a natural source, such as a plant). An ND may work with a physician or other health practitioner, referring patients to an appropriate medical specialist, such as a rheumatologist or a surgeon, as needed.

Organizations

The American Association of Naturopathic Physicians
601 Valley Street, Suite 105
Seattle, WA 98109
Phone: 206/298-0126
Fax: 206/298-0129
E-mail: aanp@usa.net
Web site: http://www.naturopathic.org
Can help you find a licensed naturopathic doctor

Bastyr University
14500 Juanita Drive NE
Kenmore, WA 98028-4966
Phone: 425/823-1300
Web site: http://www.bastyr.edu

Southwest College of Naturopathic Medicine & Health Sciences
2140 East Broadway Road
Tempe, AZ 85282
Phone: 602/858-9100
Web site: http://www.scnm.edu

National College of Naturopathic Medicine
049 SW Porter Street
Portland, OR 97201
Phone: 503/499-4343
Web site: http://www.ncnm.edu

Books

The Encyclopedia of Natural Medicine, Revised 2nd Edition, by Michael T. Murray, ND, and Joseph E. Pizzorno, ND. 1997. Rocklin, CA. Prima Publishing. Paperback. $24.95.

Formulas for Healthful Living, Second Edition, by Francis J. Brinker, ND. 1998. Eclectic Medical Publications. Paperback. $12.95.

The Natural Physician, by Mark Stengler. 1998. Alive Books. Paperback. $12.95.

What Happens in a Naturopathic Treatment

A consultation with a naturopathic doctor begins with a thorough medical history that covers all aspects of the person's lifestyle. It may also include standard diagnostic tests (such as blood and urine screenings) used in allopathic medicine. Treatment may involve any number of practices, depending on both the practitioner's particular specialty and the patient's needs. In general, the ND will suggest lifestyle changes for better health. When necessary, herbal and other medicines maybe used.

What Naturopathic Medicine Offers People with Arthritis

Naturopathic medicine, with its emphasis on nutrition and healthy lifestyles, is well-suited for treating chronic diseases such as arthritis. NDs are well-educated in nutrition and diet, and often have an expertise in botanical supplement therapies. Because naturopathic medicine has such a broad range of therapies, it can be used along with conventional – and unconventional – medicine. It may be a good choice for those who want to try complementary therapies.

However, naturopathic physicians cannot prescribe medications you may need for your arthritis, so you will want to choose an ND who will work with your physician.

Finding a Practitioner

Naturopathy is offered by a range of practitioners. It's best to consult one who is a graduate of an accredited naturopathic medical school and licensed. In 1999, 11 of 50 states (Alaska, Arizona, Connecticut, Hawaii, Maine, Montana, New Hampshire, Oregon, Utah, Vermont and Washington) and Puerto Rico had naturopathic licensing laws. In these states NDs must have graduated from a school accredited by the Council on Naturopathic Medical Education.

Also, ask about the ND's specialization to see if he or she offers practices that you wish to use.

Good Advice

- Naturopathic medicine has many strengths but is not geared to treating severe disease, and naturopathic doctors cannot prescribe medication. A reputable ND will encourage you to also consult a rheumatologist if you have RA, lupus or other severe rheumatic disease.
- Don't stop taking prescribed medications without consulting with your physician. It can be dangerous to stop some drugs suddenly.

Costs

Fees vary across the country. A first visit of one hour or so will cost $100-$200, with follow-up visits charged at $50-$75. Insurance coverage varies as well: Many companies will cover naturopathic medicine.

OSTEOPATHIC MEDICINE:
HANDS-ON THREAPY

Osteopathic medicine is usually listed with complementary therapies, but most of today's osteopathic doctors would object to that. They regard it as a mainstream medicine. Doctors of osteopathy (DOs) complete a training, certification and licensing program that is almost exactly the same as that of an allopathic medical doctor (MD). They are licensed to perform surgery and write prescriptions. They can also specialize in fields such as rheumatology, and generally do anything a medical doctor can do.

But the principles behind osteopathic medicine – and its origins – differ from allopathic medicine. Osteopathy was developed in 1872 by a Civil War surgeon named Andrew Still who became disillusioned by the limits of conventional medicine after his wife and three of his children died of spinal meningitis. He believed that mainstream medicine didn't look at the relationship between body structure and disease or utilize the body's innate ability to heal itself.

Dr. Still founded a four-year medical college that taught the allopathic medicine of his day along with his theories of healing and osteopathic manipulation. However, in spite of the emphasis on allopathic training, osteopathy was not accepted by the American Medical Association (AMA) until the 1940s. Today, osteopathic doctors (DO) are licensed in all 50 states and there are 19 osteopathic medical schools. Although some DOs specialize, most go into practice as primary care doctors.

Key Principles and Practices

The musculoskeletal system is a key element in osteopathic medicine. It makes up two-thirds of the body's mass and supports the soft tissues of the body. Osteopathic doctors believe problems with the musculoskeletal system can affect our health in many ways, and that illness can, in turn, upset the balance of this system. Another basic principle is that improved blood flow can help most illnesses or conditions, and that manipulation improves circulation. Once structural problems are corrected or eased, it's believed the body can help heal itself.

Osteopathic manipulation is most often used on soft tissues (such as muscles) around the joints and spine, but a practitioner may also use quick, strong thrusts similar to those used in chiropractic. Some osteopaths use a gentle manipulation of the bones and tissues of the skull and spine, called cranial manipulation (an offshoot of this is CranioSacral Therapy, see page 120). This very subtle therapy is used for headaches and other ills. Other practices include massage, relaxation, diet changes and exercises.

Since its beginnings, osteopathic medicine has used therapies from many traditions. Many osteopaths use therapies such as homeopathy, Chinese and Ayurvedic medicine, and natural medicines.

What Happens in an Osteopathic Treatment

A visit to a DO can be much like a visit to an MD, but it's generally more hands-on and there will be much more emphasis on body alignment and function. In addition to the usual examination and questions about your health and lifestyle, you may be asked to stand, sit and walk and be checked for flexibility, muscle strength and skeletal symmetry. The practitioner may move your limbs through range of motion and look for tender spots.

The treatment strategy will then be designed to meet your situation and diagnosis. It can involve osteopathic manipulation of your spine or joints. The practitioner may also offer – or refer you to – other therapies such as acupuncture, mind–body practices and physical therapy.

Osteopathic doctors use prescription drugs as well: In fact, if you have rheumatoid arthritis, lupus or other inflammatory arthritis, it is likely a DO will prescribe the same drugs an MD rheumatologist would recommend.

What Osteopathic Medicine Offers People with Arthritis

Osteopathy may be especially helpful to those with all kinds of arthritis, because it combines an expertise in the musculoskeletal system with a background in allopathic medicine. Some osteopathic doctors specialize in rheumatology, either as primary care doctors or as board-certified rheumatologists. These doctors use standard

RESOURCES *
OSTEOPATHIC MEDICINE

Organization
American Osteopathic Association
142 East Ontario Street
Chicago, IL 60611
Phone: 800/621-1773
E-mail: webmaster@aoc-net.org
Web site: http://www.aoa-net.org
The AOA is a professional organization. It offers patient information and referrals to osteopathic practitioners with an expertise in rheumatology.

Books
Osteopathic Medicine: An American Reformation, Third Edition, by George W. Northup, DO. 1987. Chicago, IL. American Osteopathic Association. Paperback. $6. To order, call 800/621-1773, ext. 8254.

The D.O.s : Osteopathic Medicine in America, by Norman Gevitz. 1991. Johns Hopkins University Press. Paperback. $17.95.

treatments, but can also offer hands-on medicine such as massage, stretching and manipulation to ease pain and help correct and restore function.

The practitioner can help you discover and correct patterns of movement that may be making your arthritis worse; and osteopathic manipulation after joint-replacement or other surgery may help you get moving sooner.

Many DOs practice more like MDs and will not offer as many unconventional therapies. If complementary therapies are your main interest in seeking a DO, you will need to ask about the types of treatments the doctor uses.

Finding a Practitioner

There are about 50,000 licensed DOs in the United States. They have admitting privileges to hospitals and can be found at many health maintenance organizations and clinics. Like MDs, they also specialize, so when looking for a DO, ask if he or she specializes in treating your type of arthritis. You can contact the American Osteopathic Association for a referral (see Resources).

Cautions

! A DO will be aware of the precautions to take in manipulation. However, be sure to tell him or her if you are having a flare or any increased symptoms of your disease.

Good Advice

• As in consulting any practitioner, choose someone who shares your philosophies about healing and with whom you can have a comfortable relationship.

• If you have arthritis or a musculoskeletal disorder, and prefer a DO, look for one who has expertise in rheumatology or who works closely with a rheumatologist.

Costs

Fees and insurance coverage for osteopaths are about the same as for MDs. Costs range from $50 to $100 for an office visit. An initial consultation fee can vary from $100 to $250, depending on the complexity of your condition.

CHIROPRACTIC: ALIGNING THE SPINE

If you haven't consulted a chiropractor, you probably know somebody who has. Chiropractic is the third largest health-care profession in the country, used by more than 50 million Americans a year, primarily for back or neck pain following an injury or accident.

It focuses on the manual adjustment or manipulation of the spine and probably goes back to antiquity: "bonesetters" and others who used manipulation therapy are mentioned often in medical histories. But the term and the therapy as we know it were created in Davenport, Iowa, in 1895 by a charismatic entrepreneur named Daniel David Palmer.

Palmer founded a chiropractic school in 1897. He was arrested in 1906 for practicing medicine without a license, which set off a long battle with the medical establishment. The American Medical Association (AMA) declared chiropractic quackery. But in 1987, a group of chiropractors won an anti-trust suit against the AMA. Since then, chiropractic has been increasingly accepted in conventional health care, especially for sports and other injuries. Chiropractors now serve on some hospital staffs and work with orthopaedic and neurology specialists.

Key Principles and Practices

Palmer founded chiropractic based on the theory that misalignment of vertebrae in the spine (called subluxation) is the cause of almost all diseases, and that chiropractic adjustment of the spine is the cure. The basic idea is that the nervous system, which affects the entire body and runs through the spinal column, can be blocked or damaged by problems in the spine or elsewhere in the musculoskeletal system. Thus, not only back pain but problems elsewhere, such as in the knee or wrist, could be due to a dysfunction in the spine, or could cause spinal dysfunction. When the spine is adjusted properly, the pain disappears and the body is free to heal itself.

Chiropractors complete a four-year program at one of 17 accredited chiropractic colleges. They focus mainly on musculoskeletal issues, but are also trained in general diagnostics, and in use of herbal and dietary supplements. They use a number of manual techniques, including very brief high velocity thrusts called adjustments, stretching, traction and slow manipulations of joints.

Today, there are two basic kinds of chiropractors, called "straights" and "mixers." Traditional, or "straight," chiropractors do only spinal manipulations. They don't use any other treatments, Western or alternative. Much more common are "mixers": chiropractors who use a combination of treatments and techniques, including electrical stimulation, ultrasound, homeopathy, herbal and vitamin therapies, and nutritional counseling. They may also be trained or certified in related fields, such as massage therapy, acupuncture or physical therapy.

What Happens in a Chiropractic Treatment

At your first visit, the practitioner will take a detailed medical history, and perform a physical examination to rule out any conditions that should not be treated with spinal manipulation. In some cases, the therapist may order X-rays. However, there is no need to expose yourself to the radiation (and expense) of X-rays unless a serious disease is suspected. If that's the case, you should be examined by a medical doctor before having chiropractic adjustments.

The practitioner will ask you to remove just enough clothing so he or she can examine and work on your body. You'll then sit or lie down on a table while the practitioner moves and stretches your joints, checking for misalignments. Spinal or other joint manipulation is usually done with the bare hands, but your thera-pist may use a special instrument. He or she will apply pressure in a precise spot to forcefully thrust a joint into place, or gently ease it into alignment to help restore mobility and function.

This shouldn't be painful, though sometimes you may feel a bit of discomfort during or after a manipulation. Some people feel an immediate and complete relief. You might hear a sound: It's not really your joint cracking, but air moving around in your joint during the adjustment.

The practitioner may also suggest diet changes or exercises, or use any number of other therapies such as those listed above. Your condition may need one or several treatments, but you should see some improvement fairly quickly. If you aren't any better at all after a month, chiropractic is probably not helping and you should consider other treatment options.

What Chiropractic Medicine Offers People with Arthritis

Those with joint disease should proceed with caution when considering chiropractic or other joint manipulation. Although side effects are rare for those with healthy bones and joints, manipulation could damage joints that are inflamed, diseased or weakened by osteoporosis, osteoarthritis, rheumatoid arthritis, ankylosing spondylitis and any other disease of the joints. A reputable chiropractor will not offer to use forceful manipulations for these ailments.

However, some chiropractic manipulation of knee or other joints with OA may improve function and relieve pain (Berkson). There is also some evidence that chiropractic can ease fibromyalgia symptoms: A pilot study that looked at 21 patients with fibromyalgia found that four weeks of spinal and soft tissue manipulations and stretching improved range of motion and reported pain levels (Blunt).

If you have an uncomplicated acute lower back or neck problem (in an area with no arthritis), spinal manipulation may help get you out of pain faster. Study results are mixed. In 1994, the Agency for Health Care Policy and Research recommended chiropractic as better than bed rest, traction or surgery for short-term back pain. However, a recent study showed that it was no more effective for acute back pain than physical therapy, and barely better than reading an educational booklet about back care (Cherkin). Chiropractors have challenged the design and procedures used in this study.

Millions of people find chiropractic is effective for them. If you decide to try it, be sure to tell any chiropractor you consult about your arthritis, and be sure to tell your physician about your chiropractic treatment.

Finding a Practitioner

Chiropractors are trained in four-year chiropractic colleges and are licensed in all 50 states, the District of Columbia, the U.S. Virgin Islands and Puerto Rico. A licensed chiropractor is known as a "doctor of chiropractic," and will have a DC after his or her name. They are not, however, licensed to prescribe drugs or perform surgery.

There are more than 48,000 licensed chiropractors.

You'll see chiropractors listed just about everywhere, but you will want to consult one who has experience in treating people with your kind of arthritis. You may also want to work with a chiropractor who has an added specialty such as homeopathy, massage or acupuncture. Many medical doctors and physical therapists work closely with chiropractors and can give you a referral. The organizations in Resources can also refer you to a practitioner near you.

Cautions

! If you have inflamed joints, osteoporosis or a rheumatic disease such as lupus, consult a medical doctor before you seek chiropractic treatment or any other joint manipulation.

! Be wary of practitioners who claim spinal manipulation can cure just about anything that ails you, from infections to bed wetting. So far, experts say, there are just no studies to prove this.

! If you are taking anticoagulants, be especially sure to tell the chiropractor, as these can increase bleeding or bruising.

RESOLUTION * CHIROPRACTIC

Organizations

American Chiropractic Association
1701 Clarendon Boulevard
Arlington, VA 22209
Phone: 800/986-4636
Fax: 703/243-2593
E-mail: MEMBERINFO@Amerchiro.org
Web site: http://www.amerchiro.org
Can refer to a practitioner or state chapter.

Foundation for Chiropractic Education and Research
P.O. Box 4689
Des Moines, IA 50306-4689
Phone: 800/622-6309
Web site: http://www.fcer.org
Has research on chiropractic.

Books

The Art of Healthy Living: The Consumer's Guide to Chiropractic Care, a publication of the American Chiropractic Association. Phone 800/986-4636 for free copy.

Chiropractic Library: Compassion & Expectation, by Terry A. Rondberg, DC, and Timothy J. Feuling. 1999. Chiropractic Journal. $12.95.

Good Advice

- Although studies show that spinal manipulation can help many people, not everyone – or every ill – is a good candidate for chiropractic.
- Be sure the chiropractor knows your complete health history and every medication you are taking, including supplements and vitamins.
- Be sure X-rays are absolutely necessary. A chiropractor may want a set before beginning treatment to rule out any spinal lesions or fractures, but repeat X-rays are generally not useful and expose you to unnecessary radiation.

Costs

Fees vary across the country but range from $50 to $100 or more for a first visit, less for follow-up visits. Ask the practitioner how many visits he or she thinks you will need. Most insurance companies (including Medicare) cover chiropractic and it is covered under state workers' compensation.

HOMEOPATHY: THE LAW OF SIMILARS

Homeopathy has long been practiced in Europe and was one of the most popular healing systems in the United States in the mid-19th century. By 1844, there was a homeopathic institute in the United States, thousands of homeopathic doctors, and homeopathic hospitals, pharmacies and medical schools. It faded from popularity in the 1930s but was revived again in the 1970s. Today, it ranks in the top 10 complementary therapies, and is used by medical doctors as well as naturopaths, chiropractors, herbalists, midwives and many others.

The main theory behind homeopathy is that "like cures like." Giving people miniscule amounts of materials that would cause illness in a healthy person can provoke the body of a sick person into healing the illness.

It was developed by the German physician Samuel Hahnemann in the 18th century after he discovered that the malaria drug quinine could produce malaria-like symptoms in healthy people. By testing ingredients on healthy volunteers (including himself), Hahnemann built a pharmacy of thousands of "remedies" derived from natural substances such as herbs, minerals and animal products, all used in very tiny amounts. His system very quickly became popular in Europe, Asia and America as millions of people were drawn to the concept of treating illness with minute amounts of natural ingredients.

Key Principles and Practices

Hahnemann's interest in homeopathy – and a reason for its popularity – was a reaction to the crude and ineffective mainstream medicine of the time. He believed living things have a vital life force that, when stimulated by the subtle energy of the correct remedy, will restore and maintain health. The vital force concept is similar to that of prana in ayurveda or qi in Chinese medicine. Homeopathic medicines don't try to ease symptoms; rather, they "provoke" the body to respond and thus heal and strengthen itself.

Diagnosis focuses on the symptoms rather than a disease, and treatment consists of giving remedies that will create the same symptoms. "Classical" homeopaths identify a patient's "constitutional type" and choose remedies to treat that. Nonclassical homeopaths, which are more common in the United States, give remedies based on the symptom.

Hahnemann believed that the weaker the remedy, the stronger the reaction: Therefore remedies are highly diluted, sometimes so diluted that not a single molecule of the original material remains in the solution or tablet. No one can explain how this works – or how

Organization

National Center for Homeopathy
801 North Fairfax Street, Suite 306
Alexandria, VA 22314
Phone: 703/548-7790
E-mail: nchinfo@igc.org
Web site: http://www.homeopathic.org/index.html
Publishes the magazine *Homeopathy Today*, and has a list of certifying organizations and a directory of practitioners.

Books

Everybody's Guide to Homeopathic Medicines: Effective Remedies for You and Your Family, by Stephen Cummings, MD, and Dana Ullman, MPH. 1997. New York. Putnam Publishing. Paperback. $16.95.

Healing with Homeopathy: The Complete Guide, by Wayne B. Jonas, MD, and Jennifer Jacobs, MD, MPH. 1996. New York. Warner Books. Hardcover. $24.95.

The Consumer's Guide to Homeopathy: The Definitive Resource for Understanding Homeopathic Medicine and Making It Work for You, by Dana Ullman, MPH. 1996. New York. JP Tarcher. Paperback. $13.95.

Web site

Dana Ullman's Web site has articles on homeopathy.
http://www.homeopathic.com

---

it could work. One theory is that the molecules of the remedy substance leave a kind of memory or "frequency" in the water as they disappear, and that the body responds to that. However, this hasn't been proved.

What Happens in a Homeopathy Treatment

The first consultation with a homeopath takes an hour or more, during which the practitioner will ask about your health, lifestyle, preferences and symptoms. He or she will then choose, from thousands of remedies, the one most likely to fit your symptoms and type. You may also get advice on lifestyle and nutrition.

The remedy may be in the form of a tincture, tablet or cream and might be available at the practitioner's office or through a health food or drug store. Most likely, you'll be given tiny tablets to dissolve under your tongue.

(Remedies are classified as over-the-counter drugs, and regulated like other OTCs such as aspirin.) As you use the remedy, you'll be asked to note any changes or reactions. Sometimes, symptoms worsen dramatically but briefly before they begin to get better.

A classical homeopath will give one remedy at a time, looking for a perfect fit. Practitioners of other therapies (such as chiropractic, naturopathy and so on) may give a homeopathic remedy along with other treatments or herbs. The treatment is checked in follow-up visits a month or two later. Acute ailments such as the flu or an infection may clear up with one dose, while chronic conditions such as arthritis may take many treatments.

What Homeopathy Offers People With Arthritis

It's hard to say if homeopathy does anything for any kind of arthritis. A 1998 meta-analysis (Linde) that looked at many homeopathic studies concluded that it has clinical effects that are not completely due to placebo: On average, patients were more than twice as likely to have a benefit from homeopathic remedies as from a placebo. However, there was not enough evidence to show homeopathy was effective for any one condition.

A 1980 double-blind, placebo-controlled trial of 23 people with rheumatoid arthritis found those using homeopathic remedies had a significant improvement in pain, stiffness and grip strength compared to those taking a placebo (Gibson). More recently, fibromyalgia patients in a randomized, placebo-controlled trial had a 25 percent reduction of tender spots (Fisher). But other studies showed it was no better than placebo for those with OA (Shipley) or RA (Andrade). Proponents say these studies were not well-done, and that homeopathy has been used successfully on animals, so it has more than a placebo effect.

Homeopathic remedies may be worth a try, especially if conventional medicines are not working well for you. The remedies are so diluted that treatments are unlikely to do any harm, and many people say they find relief through homeopathy.

Finding a Practitioner

Homeopathy practitioners are not licensed or regulated uniformly, so there is a wide range of expertise. Three states have homeopathic licensing laws: MDs and DOs practicing homeopathy in Arizona or Nevada, and MDs practicing in Connecticut must be licensed by the state homeopathic licensing board.

Many health professionals practice homeopathy, including medical and osteopathic doctors, chiropractors, veterinarians, dentists, nurse practitioners, physician assistants, acupuncturists, and certified nurse midwives. Naturopathic physicians study homeopathy as part of naturopathic medical school. It's also practiced by people with no medical training at all. Moreover, the level of competence in homeopathy often has little to do with any certification or medical training.

Your best bet is to find someone who has been through a homeopathic training or certification program. Some organizations list members by state. However, not all practitioners are members (see Resources). Ask health professionals and friends for referrals to a practitioner with experience in treating your kind of musculoskeletal disorder.

You can also self-treat for minor ailments like colds or the flu: Many pharmacies and health food stores have homeopathic remedies labeled for the conditions they treat.

Cautions

! There are few risks with homeopathy, because the remedies are so diluted. The remedies are regulated as over-the-counter drugs by the FDA.

! Homeopathy should not be used alone to treat severe disease or life-threatening illness. Be sure to consult a physician.

! Some homeopaths claim that conventional drugs can interfere with the homeopathic treatments. However, don't stop any prescribed medication without consulting your doctor: It can be dangerous to stop some drugs suddenly.

Costs

Fees range from $100 to $400 for the first consultation and from $50 to $100 for follow-up visits. The remedies are inexpensive: They generally cost $5-$15.

Homeopathy is covered by some health insurance, especially when treatments are provided by a physician or other health-care professional.

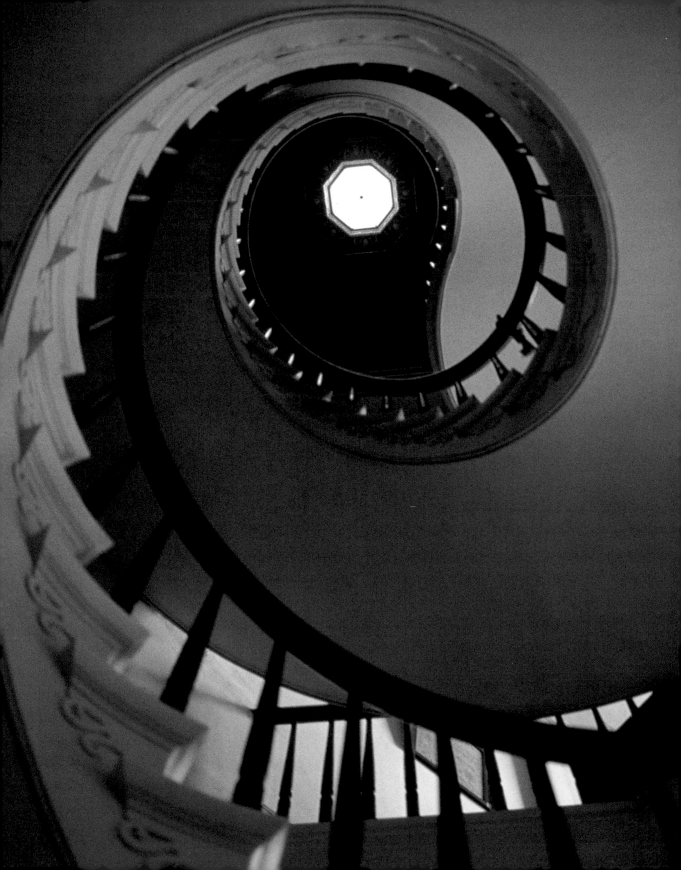

Mind, Body
And Spirit

CREATING A UNITED FRONT

It's no secret that your mental health is connected to your physical health. When you don't feel well physically, you don't feel well mentally, and vice versa. And when you have a chronic illness, the mind–body connection becomes even more apparent. Pain and sickness make you vulnerable to stress, depression and anxiety. These negative emotions then turn up the volume on pain and increase symptoms. Sometimes, it can feel as if your life has spun out of control, and that you are caught in an endless cycle of physical and emotional pain.

Mind–body medicine can help you gain control of your life again. It focuses on the powerful ways in which emotional, mental, social and spiritual factors interact with your body and affect your health. It offers therapies you can learn to use yourself to improve your physical and emotional well-being. The practice of these therapies has been shown to restore a sense of self-control and self-worth that can contribute greatly to your overall health.

By connecting your mind and body through the techniques discussed in this chapter, you may ease your symptoms, help break the cycle of pain and depression, and improve the quality of your life.

Making the Mind–Body Connection

In ancient times, the role of the mind and spirit in physical health was well-accepted.

Many of the practices discussed in this chapter – such as meditation, visualization and hypnosis – were part of healing. But since the scientific revolution, Western medicine has tended to see the body and mind as separate entities. The body is often thought of as a kind of machine, and the role of thoughts and emotions has been downplayed.

A few decades ago, researchers began to look more closely at the complicated interconnection of the body and mind. Researchers had long known about the powerful effects of mind over body in something called the placebo effect. Placebo (which means "I will please" in Latin) is an inactive treatment or pill scientists often use when conducting studies. One group of patients gets the treatment or drug being tested, and another gets a placebo. Then the results are compared to see if the treatment being studied has an effect greater than placebo. About 30 percent of people getting an inactive treatment respond as though it were the real thing.

Researchers didn't see much value in this result at first, nor did they know how to explain it. Often, the effect diminished or disappeared as soon as patients learned they weren't getting the real treatment. Generally, the placebo effect was seen as a sign of impressionability or even weakness in people who could be swayed by the power of suggestion.

Researchers began learning more about the connection between stress and disease. Studies

Empowerment: Taking Control of Your Life

Gaining a sense of control over your chronic illness can be a key factor in decreasing pain and depression. You can gain the confidence to manage your condition through educational and empowerment programs. One study reviewed controlled trials of patient education programs compared with trials of NSAID treatments for patients with osteoarthritis and rheumatoid arthritis. The authors found the education programs gave 20 percent to 30 percent greater pain relief for all; and for those with rheumatoid arthritis, 40 percent greater improvement in function and 60 percent to 80 percent better reduction of tender joint counts (Superio-Cabuslay).

The Arthritis Self-Help Course created by Kate Lorig, DrPH, RN, of the Stanford Arthritis Center is one such successful program. The six-week series of classes includes basic disease information, relaxation techniques for pain and stress management, an overview of arthritis medications, design of a comprehensive exercise program, techniques for coping with depression and other problem-solving strategies.

The course is recommended and given by the Arthritis Foundation. You can find an Arthritis Self-Help Course being held near you by calling your local Arthritis Foundation, or the national office at 800/283-7800.

RESOURCES ✳

The book that accompanies the course can also be used on its own.

Books
The Arthritis Helpbook: A Tested Self-Management Program for Coping with Arthritis and Fibromyalgia, Fifth Edition by Kate Lorig, DrPH, RN, and James F. Fries, MD. Reading, MA: Perseus, 2000. Paperback.

It is also available in Spanish as:
Como Convivir con su Artritis by Virginia Gonzalez. Palo Alto, CA: Bull Publishing Co, 1997. $12.95.

showed that stress adds to risk of high blood pressure and heart disease; contributes to irritable bowel disease, skin problems (psoriasis and eczema) and allergies; and undermines the immune system, leaving us more vulnerable to infections and, some say, even cancer. It also magnifies the effects of pain, anxiety and depression.

Mind–Body Therapies

The therapies below used in mind–body medicine can show you how to reduce pain, depression and physical and mental stress, and improve your overall health.

- **Biofeedback** uses electronic monitors to teach you how to use your mind to affect many body functions. It has been shown to help relieve headache, pain and Raynaud's phenomenon.

- **Meditation** is an ancient practice that develops calmness, concentration and insight, and has been shown to relieve pain, stress and depression.

- **Visualization and guided imagery** use the power of your imagination to relieve pain, promote relaxation and change behavior patterns. These techniques can have many effects but are most used to relieve stress and anxiety and promote healing.

- **Hypnosis** is a technique to alter your consciousness that helps focus attention and foster relaxation.

- **Relaxation exercises** help make you aware of tension and show you how to release it. **Breathing exercises** use the connection between breath and emotions to teach relaxation and to energize. **Body scan** and **progressive muscle relaxation** bring a non-judging connection to the body, increasing awareness of physical sensations and teaching muscle-by-muscle relaxation.

- **Stress reduction and relaxation** programs combine many of these techniques along with moving meditations such as yoga, tai chi and qi gong (see Moving Medicine, page 97).

Much of our stress is due to an out-dated fight-or-flight response, a hangover from a more primitive era when we needed rapid instinctive responses to fight off attackers, or outrun them. It's still useful in a crisis, and small doses can fire us up for a new experience or energize us for competitive sports. The trouble is, our hectic culture is full of false alarms that tend to push our fight-or-flight button inappropriately. Our bodies are often on red alert, primed to do battle or flee – with no one to fight and nowhere to go.

Many people don't know how to relax – or even know that they are in an almost constant state of tension. Chronic pain especially can set up a perpetual state of physical and mental tension, and unrelenting stress is like running all of your systems as hard and fast as they will go. Eventually, the systems begin to break down. In a sense, it's like the placebo effect in reverse, with the mind generating negative responses such as stress, anxiety and depression.

These observations began to explain something that had long puzzled doctors: Why patients with the same chronic illness often had such different symptoms, levels of disability and experience of pain. Research began to show that emotional and psychological factors are connected to the amount of pain and disability a person experiences, and that mind–body therapies can significantly affect the level of illness.

This prompted a whole new area of study and treatment called "behavioral medicine" that looks at the effects of behavior, thoughts and emotions on medical conditions such as arthritis and chronic pain. Cognitive–behavioral therapy to help patients become aware of and change mental attitudes was shown to help many (Parker 1). Cognitive–behavioral therapists also became increasingly interested in the "alternative" mind–body practices, and began including them in therapy.

Today an increasing number of doctors treating chronic illness are looking at the emotional, social and behavioral aspects of their patients as well as their physical health. Stress reduction and relaxation programs that teach mind–body techniques are offered at many hospitals across the county.

Education programs, such as the Arthritis Self-Help Course sponsored by the Arthritis Foundation (see Empowerment, page 55) also play an important role in health.

Researchers continue to discover more about the effects of the mind and body on each other. Psychoneuroimmunology is a branch of medicine that studies the interactions of the mind (psycho), the neurological system (neuro) and the immune system (immunology). Our very cells may "feel" emotions: Chemical messengers carry information and emotions from our brains to cells throughout our bodies. When we say "I feel that in my gut," we may be speaking the literal truth.

Science is also taking a new look at the old placebo effect. Herbert Benson, MD, of the Mind–Body Institute at Harvard suggests that doctors harness the power of belief and replace the term "placebo effect" with the more positive concept of "remembered wellness" (Benson). Whatever it's called, the phenomenon is nothing to scoff at: A review by Benson found it accounted for beneficial clinical results in 60 to 90 percent of diseases.

Scientific Evidence

So far, no one has shown these therapies can help grow new cartilage or reverse the

Many universities now have departments or centers involved in complementary medicine or mind–body therapies. Ask about programs at a university or college near you.

Organizations

The Mind–Body Medical Institute
Division of Behavioral Medicine
Beth Israel Deaconess Medical Center
110 Francis Street, Suite 1A
Boston MA 02215
Phone: 617/632-9525
Web site: http://www.mindbody.harvard.edu
Has information about mind–body programs for different medical conditions, as well as referral to a program near you.

Stress Reduction Clinic
Center for Mindfulness in Medicine, Health Care and Society
University of Massachusetts Memorial Healthcare
Worcester, MA 01655
Phone: 508/856-2656
Provides information about mindfulness and stress reduction, as well as referral to a program near you.

Center for Mind Body Medicine
5225 Connecticut Avenue NW, Suite 414
Washington, DC 20015
Phone: 202/966-7338
E-mail: cmbm@mindspring.com
Web site: http://www.healthy.net/othersites/mindbody/index.html

Books
Anatomy of an Illness as Perceived by the Patient, by Norman Cousins. 1995. New York. W.W. Norton & Company. Hardcover. $18.95.

Full Catastrophe Living: Using the Wisdom of Your Body and Mind to Face Stress, Pain and Illness, by Jon Kabat-Zinn, PhD. 1991. New York. Dell Publishing. Paperback. $15.95.

Healing and the Mind, by Bill Moyers. 1995. New York. Doubleday & Company, Inc. Paperback. $19.95. Also available on audio tape. Adapted from the PBS television series (see below).

Mind Body Medicine: How to Use Your Mind for Better Health, edited by Daniel Goleman. 1995. Consumer Reports Books. Paperback. $11.95.

Minding the Body, Mending the Mind, by Joan Borysenko. 1988. New York. Bantam Books, Inc. Paperback. $14.95.

The Miracle of Mindfulness: A Manual on Meditation, by Thich Nhat Hanh. 1988. Boston, MA. Beacon Press. Paperback. $12.

Molecules of Emotion: Why You Feel the Way You Feel, by Candace B. Pert and Deepak Chopra. 1999. New York. Simon & Schuster. Hardcover. $25.

The Wellness Book: The Comprehensive Guide to Maintaining Health and Treating Stress-Related Illness, by Herbert Benson and E. Stuart. 1993. Fireside. Paperback. $15.

Wherever You Go, There You Are: Mindfulness Meditation in Everyday Life, by Jon Kabat-Zinn, PhD. 1994. New York. Hyperion. Paperback. $13.95.

Why Zebras Don't Get Ulcers: An Updated Guide to Stress, Stress-Related Diseases, and Coping, by Robert M. Sapolsky. 1998. W.H. Freeman & Co. Paperback. $14.95.

Web Site
The Transcendental Meditation Program Guide to Transcendental Medicine
http://www.tm.org

Audio Tapes
Guided Body Scan Meditation and Yoga 1 & 2, by Jon Kabat-Zinn, PhD. Narrates a relaxation session and a gentle yoga sequence used in the Stress Reduction Program at the University of Massachusetts. Available at some health centers and bookstores. Also available by writing Stress Reduction Tapes, P.O. Box 547, Lexington, MA 02420. Order online at http://www.mindfulnesstapes.com The two-tape set is $20. Add $2 for handling.

Molecules of Emotion: Why You Feel the Way You Feel, by Candace B. Pert. 1997. New York. Simon & Schuster. $18.

Videotape
Healing and the Mind, by Bill Moyers. A PBS television series available on video at many public libraries. The segment that describes the University of Massachusetts Stress Reduction and Relaxation Program is called "Healing from Within."

joint damage of rheumatoid arthritis and osteoarthritis. But mind–body practices have been proven to significantly relieve many of the symptoms such as pain, stress and depression that come with arthritis and related disorders (Bradley, Buckelew). A 1996 National Institutes of Health Technology Assessment Panel on Integration of Behavioral and Relaxation Approaches into the Treatment of Chronic Pain and Insomnia found strong evidence for relaxation techniques and hypnosis in reducing chronic pain. A recent review of mind–body medicine and arthritis in the *Rheumatic Disease Clinics of North America* concluded that the scientific evidence shows these therapies provide significant symptom relief and improvements in disability and well-being (Broderick).

Expert Opinion

These therapies are low cost, non-drug, noninvasive, have very few or no side effects, and can contribute to major changes in well-being. They are worth trying. However, these techniques don't work equally well for everyone. They require both a commitment of time and, often, lifestyle changes.

Start by choosing the style or type of mind–body program that appeals to you. Some may be more effective than others: They are all doors into the same room, so you need to find the "door" that feels right for you. Descriptions of the most popular techniques

Helping Your Arthritis with the Write Stuff

Sometimes, it really seems to help to just let your feelings out. Now it turns out that writing about what ails you actually could help your arthritis.

A study has found that writing about stressful experiences improved the health of people with mild to moderately severe rheumatoid arthritis or asthma. Rheumatoid arthritis patients in the study averaged a 28 percent decrease in overall disease symptoms. Their asthma counterparts had a 19 percent decrease (Smyth).

They didn't even have to write very long to get these results. Participants were asked to write continuously, without regard to spelling or even content, for 20 minutes on three consecutive days. Those in the experimental group were asked to write about the most stressful experience they ever had. Some of the topics that people chose included death of a loved one, relationship problems and seeing or being in a life-threatening accident. The control group, which showed little change on average, was asked to write about plans for the day.

The beneficial results showed up for asthma patients two weeks after the experiment, but the arthritis patients didn't show improvement until the four-month follow-up. Other studies have shown that people who express their emotions in writing improve their health outcomes, and even increase their immune function. Many have also found relief in keeping journals or writing letters that are never sent.

If you want to try writing it out, here are some resources.

RESOURCES ✳ WRITING

Organizations
Intensive Journal Program
Dialogue House
80 East 11th Street, Suite 305
New York, NY 10003
Phone: 800/221-5844 or 212/673-5880
E-mail: info@intensivejournal.org
Web site: http://www.intensivejournal.org

Center for Journal Therapy
12477 West Cedar Drive, #102
Lakewood, CO 80228
Phone: 888/421-2298
E-mail: journaldoc@aol.com
Web site: http://www.journaltherapy.com

Books
At a Journal Workshop: Writing to Access the Power of the Unconscious and Evoke Creative Ability (Inner Workbook), by Ira Progoff. New York: JP Tarcher, 1992. Paperback. $15.95.

Journal to the Self: 22 Paths to Personal Growth, by Kathleen Adams. New York: Warner Books, 1990. Paperback. $12.99.

Toward Healthy Living: A Wellness Journal. Atlanta: Arthritis Foundation, 1997. Spiral-bound. $14.95.

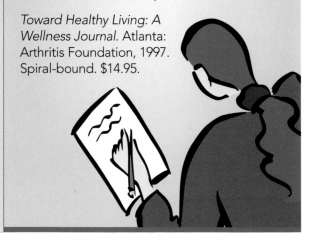

follow, beginning with the meditation section. The Resources sections list sources for more information.

Cautions

! Beware of those who say your disease is caused by your mind or your emotions, or who tells you that your attitude is keeping you from getting well. This is incorrect. Although your mind and body are connected, the life process is much more complicated than that. Such practitioners can be dangerous to your health, and they are sure to add to your stress. Stay away from them.

! If you are being treated for anxiety or other psychological conditions, talk to your therapist before you try meditation or any of the mind–body techniques involving self-analysis or introspection.

! Be aware that these techniques tap into the mind and emotions, and may bring up powerful feelings. Most often, these are feelings of peace and relaxation. But you may also experience sadness or even tears. If strong emotions continue to surface, you may want to seek counseling.

Good Advice

• Be sure to find a qualified practitioner. Although mind–body practices are offered by health professionals such as psychologists, social workers and psychiatrists, anybody can hang out a shingle and claim to be a therapist. Ask about training and certification. Seek out practitioners from an area hospital or clinic, or get a referral from a well-established professional organization.

• Reactions to mind–body therapies are individual. Not every technique may work for you. Don't feel like a failure if these techniques don't seem to help you. There are plenty of therapies to try.

MEDITATION

In just a few decades, meditation has gone from a counter-culture oddity to an accepted therapy with a valuable role in the treatment of many chronic ailments.

Meditation has its roots in our earliest religions. Since antiquity, it's been part of just about every world religion, from Christianity to Zen Buddhism. Spiritual seekers use meditation to attain a state of enlightenment, peace or a closeness with God. Yet studies show you can get many benefits from practicing meditation without any religious intention whatsoever.

Basically, meditation involves using any of a number of awareness practices to focus and quiet the mind and body. The techniques, which have been practiced for thousands of years, involve sitting in a quiet place and focusing your attention on an object, thought or sensation. This can be a sound, a holy phrase, your own breathing or bodily sensations, or an image. In the West, prayer is the best-known meditation practice (see Prayer and Spirituality, page 89).

In the late 19th century, Asian meditation practices were introduced to the West along with yoga and Indian Buddhism. But meditation didn't become well-known until the 1960s when celebrities such as the Beatles began practicing transcendental meditation with the Indian yogi Maharishi Mahesh. Around the same time, scientists began to study Asian monks for their ability to control body functions. Research confirmed that long-time meditators could affect many physical functions, including heart rate, blood pressure, and levels of stress chemicals. Herbert Benson, MD, a Harvard University professor studying the effects of meditation, demystified this process for Americans. His research showed anyone could reap the benefits of what he called "the relaxation response" by simply sitting in a quiet place and concentrating on any phrase or sound, such as the word "one." It is the practice, and not a specific technique or intent, that brings about the relaxation response, he said.

There are many ways to practice meditation. Some involve turning inward to concentrate on the silent repetition of a prayer or a holy phrase (a mantra), a sound, or the rhythm of your own breathing. Transcendental meditation uses a mantra, for example. These are known as concentration practices because they cultivate the focus of "one-pointed" attention.

How to Meditate

Choose a quiet place and a time when you won't be disturbed. It's important to find a posture that's comfortable for you. Many meditators sit cross-legged on a flat pillow on the floor because this is a very stable posture to sit for long periods of time. However, if you have arthritis affecting your knees, hips or back, this may not be comfortable for you. Try sitting in a chair with your back supported and feet flat on the ground. Try not to move or fidget because it interferes with concentration. But if you are in pain, don't suffer: Adjust your position as you must.

If your back or joints are hurting so much you can't sit still for 20 minutes, there are alternatives. You can lie down on your back for meditation, but you may fall asleep as you relax. Or you can do a walking meditation, or split the time between sitting and walking. Choose a place to walk where you won't be disturbed or have to worry about obstacles. Plan a path around a room or series of rooms in your house, or outside around the yard.

Begin to meditate by quieting your body with a few deep, relaxing breaths. Bring your attention to the word, phrase or object you are using for focus, and gently hold it there. Don't try too hard, or you'll remain tense. Let your thoughts and feelings drift by. Don't get involved in them. Don't judge yourself or your feelings. Just keep bringing your attention gently back to your focus each time the mind wanders.

As time passes, you may feel yourself relaxing and becoming peaceful. Or you may find it agonizing to remain still: Your legs may ache or your mind may be racing with thoughts, or you may be bored. This is all normal, and fine. See if you can just sit there, observing and accepting moment-to-moment whatever arises. Eventually, you will be less prone to distraction; but it's the process that's important.

At the end of the session, you might take a few deeper breaths and wait a minute or so before doing anything else or even standing up. You may be surprised at how calm and rested you feel.

Another group of meditation practices cultivates "mindfulness": a non-judgmental awareness of the present moment. These practices start by cultivating a one-pointed focus (such as on your breathing) and then expand the field to include awareness of the thoughts, emotions or changing sensations in the body. This approach is taught in many stress reduction programs modeled on the Stress Reduction and Relaxation Clinic at the University of Massachusetts, where it is called "mindfulness-based stress reduction."

In all meditation practices, the thoughts or feelings that arise during meditation are allowed to come and go. When attention wanders, it is brought gently back to the meditation object or field of attention.

The techniques for meditation are simple, but they are not easy for everyone. It takes discipline to remain still, physically and mentally, and not react to all of the stimuli in the world and in your own mind and body. This stillness is at the core of meditation and the source of its many benefits.

What Happens in a Meditation Session

Many people meditate for 20 minutes once or twice a day, but some meditate for 45 minutes to an hour a day or go on long meditation retreats to deepen their practice. For a beginner, even 10 minutes a day will reap benefits. You can meditate alone or in a group. Some types may work better for you than others. You may decide to meditate for relaxation alone, or you might be interested in exploring its spiritual dimensions. Either way, it's helpful to have some instruction from a teacher who can guide you through the process and answer questions that may come up as you practice. However, you can learn meditation quite well from books or tapes. Many people attend a few classes, and then meditate at home alone.

Meditation gives most benefit when done daily: That is why it's called a "practice." Some find it helpful to join others in a meditation session once a week.

Scientific Evidence

Meditation has been well-studied, and research shows that regular meditation can profoundly affect physical processes and benefit your overall health. It can significantly relieve chronic pain and anxiety, and it is particularly effective for fibromyalgia, especially when combined with other mind–body techniques. In a 1993 uncontrolled study of 77 patients with fibromyalgia who participated in a 10-week meditation-based relaxation program, all showed some improvement and 51 percent had moderate to marked improvement (Kaplan).

A number of studies from the University of Massachusetts Medical Center have shown that mindfulness-based stress reduction provides substantial and lasting reductions in pain and anxiety among people with chronic pain. An uncontrolled study of 51 chronic pain patients who had not improved with conventional medical care found that half showed a pain reduction of 50 percent or more following a 10-week meditation-based program (Kabat-Zinn 1). In another uncontrolled study, 60 percent of a group of 225 meditators with chronic pain continued to show some improvement four years after the program (Kabat-Zinn 2).

Meditation is often combined with other mind–body techniques. An uncontrolled study of 28 women with fibromyalgia found that an eight-week program of mindfulness meditation combined with qi gong and pain management techniques gave significant improvement in pain threshold, depression, coping and function (Singh). A follow-up study showed these results lasted for at least four months after the program ended (Creamer).

Transcendental meditation has been studied mostly by the Maharishi International University, the organization that teaches and markets it. The methodology of some of these studies has been questioned. However, one showed that regular transcendental meditators used fewer medical services and made fewer doctor visits (Orme-Johnson). Another showed that during and after meditation, regular meditators had a decrease in their levels of the stress chemical cortisol (Jevning).

Expert Opinion

Meditation is a useful, safe and low-cost therapy for many symptoms of arthritis and related diseases, particularly stress, depression and pain. Meditation is generally safe, especially when practiced for 45 minutes or less a day. But the practice can tap deep into the subconscious and may uncover suppressed emotions, so it's important to choose an instructor with care.

Some people will find it difficult to be still long enough to learn or practice the techniques. Some might be uncomfortable with the spiritual aspects of some approaches and may do better with other practices such as relaxation exercises or biofeedback.

Finding a Practitioner

Meditation instruction is not certified or licensed on a national level. It's taught by various spiritual organizations and yoga or meditation centers; by psychologists and other mental health professionals; and at an increasing number of hospitals, medical centers and clinics. Be sure to ask about training and qualifications. Mental health professionals are, of course, licensed to do therapy, and some use meditation. Instructors in spiritual organizations are often appointed after completing an apprenticeship with a master teacher.

You may see advertisements for meditation retreats or workshops. Some are sponsored by churches or other religious groups or by new-age

Many types of meditation and organizations offer instruction. See the list of general mind–body resources on page 58. A "new age" bookstore in your area may be able to direct you to local resources.

Organizations

Insight Meditation Society
1230 Pleasant Street
Barre, MA 01500
Phone: 978/355-4378
E-mail: david@dharma.org
Web site: http://www.dharma.org

The Transcendental Meditation Program
Phone: 888/532-7686
E-mail: info@tm.org
Web site: http://www.tm.org

Books

Heal Thy Self: Lessons on Mindfulness in Medicine, by Saki Santorelli. 1999. New York. Crown Publishing Group. Hardcover. $23.

The Meditative Mind: Varieties of Meditative Experience, by Daniel Goleman and Ram Dass. 1996. New York. JP Tarcher. Paperback. $11.95.

The Miracle of Mindfulness: A Manual of Meditation, by Thich Nhat Hanh. 1996. Boston, Beacon Press. Hardcover. $17.

Science of Being and Art of Living: Transcendental Meditation, by Maharishi Mahesh Yogi. Reprint edition 1994. Meridian Books. Paperback. $16.

Web Sites

The Insight Meditation Center Online
Has links to several meditation centers
http://www.dharma.org

Complete Guide to the Transcendental Meditation Program
http://www.tm.org

Audio Tape

Mindfulness Meditation Practice Tapes
Stress Reduction Tapes
P.O. Box 547
Lexington, MA 02420
Web site: http://www.mindfulnesstapes.com
Series 2 is a five-tape set, sold only as a complete set, of guided meditation. $35 plus $4 for shipping/handling.

spiritual centers. These can vary widely in quality, so check out the organizers before you isolate yourself with strangers for a weekend or longer. You might be most comfortable – and secure – at your local hospital, health or community center learning a nonreligious meditation through a stress reduction program.

Good Advice

- If one kind of meditation doesn't seem to work for you, there are several others you can try. It does help to get instruction in the beginning.
- Trust your instincts: If a meditation instructor or process makes you uncomfortable, stop and leave.
- Don't get hung up on correct postures for sitting. The important point is to meditate. If pain from arthritis prevents you from assuming the classic position, just do what feels best and enjoy the meditation rather than suffer the position.

Costs

Fees for meditation courses vary. Some meditation centers offer courses free of charge or for a donation, whereas other organizations charge from $50 to $600. Yoga or meditation centers often have free daily or weekly group meditations. Most stress reduction programs teach meditation and other mind–body techniques. These programs cost $150 and up for a six-to10-week session, and may be covered by your health insurer. Ask your doctor for a referral. Mental health professionals who teach meditation usually charge the same as a regular session: $40–$125 per hour.

BIOFEEDBACK

Biofeedback is a marriage of modern technology and ancient meditation techniques. It's the use of electronic instruments to measure body functions and feed this information back to you so you learn to control them. With practice, you can learn to change just about any body process that can be measured, such as your pulse and blood pressure. You can learn to relax tense muscles to ease fibromyalgia pain, and to increase circulation and raise the temperature in your hands to relieve Raynaud's discomfort.

Biofeedback can be particularly useful because it teaches people to become aware of and control a specific body part or function, such as relaxing one muscle in your neck or raising the temperature in your hands. Until a few decades ago, most Western scientists thought these functions were involuntary, and that it was impossible to consciously control them. Reports of yoga and other meditation masters who could slow their heart rates or suspend breathing were considered phony. Then research proved these masters could indeed affect involuntary functions. Further study showed that ordinary people who had proper training could use biofeedback to relieve chronic pain, stress, anxiety, muscle tension and gastrointestinal disorders (see Scientific Evidence). It is now so accepted that many consider it to be a mainstream therapy.

What Happens in a Biofeedback Session

In a biofeedback session, sensors are painlessly attached to the part of your body that's being monitored and then connected to an electronic instrument, such as a computer. Some sensors are held in place with a temporary glue that wipes off. One type slips over your finger like a cigar band. The instruments might read your skin temperature, electrical signals produced by your muscles, your heart rate, or your brain waves.

The practitioner will teach you some mind–body techniques such as visualization or relaxation to influence your subconscious (or autonomic) body processes. As you practice these mental techniques, the instruments feed back the effects your thoughts are having on your body with sound, light or other signals. Some use a computer screen with graphs or charts that change as your body functions change. Eventually, you will learn what mental techniques to use to get the physical effect you want, and will be able to do these on your own without the equipment.

The number of sessions needed varies with your situation: It can take a few sessions, or

20 sessions for you to learn how to relieve your symptoms. There are devices and computer programs you can get to practice biofeedback at home. An inexpensive tool to measure skin temperature changes can help those with Raynaud's learn to raise hand temperature. It's best to have a session with a biofeedback practitioner and ask for advice before you buy equipment to be sure you're getting what you need.

Scientific Evidence

Biofeedback has been shown to improve function and relieve pain and stress for several conditions, especially when combined with relaxation and other mind–body therapies.

A two-phase controlled study of patients with rheumatoid arthritis found relaxation and biofeedback gave significant improvements in pain, tension and sleep patterns when compared to physiotherapy (Achterberg). An 18-month review of rheumatoid arthritis patients who used biofeedback and other behavioral modification therapies showed they had reduced clinic visits, days hospitalized and lower medical costs (Young).

An uncontrolled study looked at the effects of biofeedback and relaxation training on eight children with high pain levels from juvenile rheumatoid arthritis. Results showed that half reported at least a 25 percent decrease in pain. At a six-month follow-up, slightly more of the children reported at least

RESORCE *
BIOFEEDBACK

Biofeedback Certification Institute of America
10200 West 44th Avenue, Suite 304
Wheat Ridge, CO 80023
Phone: 303/420-2902
Certifies practitioners. Send a stamped, self-addressed envelope for information.

a 25 percent reduction in pain (Lavigne).

Several studies and case reports show biofeedback helped those with Raynaud's phenomenon by teaching them to raise hand temperatures and increase blood circulation. One group of researchers reviewed the records of 23 patients with varying degrees of Raynaud's who were trained in biofeedback (Yocum). All had higher baseline finger temperatures after biofeedback training. Those who also had scleroderma or lupus had the greatest temperature increases. Improvements lasted for a year after the treatment and four of the study participants were able to raise their hand temperatures 18 months after the training ended.

Expert Opinion

Biofeedback can be a valuable treatment for chronic pain, tension and Raynaud's phenomenon. Once you've learned the technique, you can use it just about anywhere without the monitors. There are no side effects from biofeedback.

Finding a Practitioner

Biofeedback is used by many health professionals including medical doctors, physical therapists and psychologists. In many states it is not regulated; some states do limit its practice to health professionals. Thousands of biofeedback practitioners are certified by the Biofeedback Certification Institute of America, which can supply referrals (see Resources). Many practitioners are listed in the Yellow Pages: Be sure to ask about certification and training. However, your doctor may be the best source for referral to a biofeedback program, as he or she will want to know about your treatments.

Also, treatments or equipment prescribed by your doctor may be covered by insurance.

Good Advice

- Biofeedback is most effective when used with other mind–body techniques.
- The amount of time it takes to make biofeedback work varies from person to person. Be sure to give it a long enough trial.

Costs

Fees range from about $40 to $150 or more a session. Health insurance coverage varies, but biofeedback sessions may be reimbursed if you have a physician's prescription. However, once you've mastered the techniques you can use them anytime to help yourself. You can lower costs by having a few sessions with a practitioner and then buying some equipment for home use.

VISUALIZATION AND GUIDED IMAGERY

The power of your imagination can help you cope with many arthritis symptoms. With visualization or guided imagery you can ease pain and anxiety, develop a more positive self-image, and boost your body's healing ability. A practitioner guides you through the exercises, or you can learn to practice these techniques yourself with the help of audio tapes.

The terms visualization and imagery are often used interchangeably because they are so closely related. In visualization, you vividly imagine the outcome that you want, or mentally take yourself there. If you are in pain, for example, you might go to a place of peace and relaxation, or imagine yourself moving without pain. In guided imagery, a practitioner helps you reach a state of deep relaxation or a trance and then guides you through an exercise or gives you suggestions to help you reach your goals.

These techniques have long been used to control pain, overcome phobias, treat addictions, and to help athletes and others improve their performance. Many mental health professionals use them, and they are often part of psychotherapy, biofeedback, stress reduction and relaxation programs.

Visualization and guided imagery are safe, non-drug techniques that have significantly helped some people cope with a range of ailments. They also contribute to a positive self-image and can be used to motivate you to a happier and more active lifestyle.

What Happens in a Visualization Session

Visualization techniques are taught in group or private sessions. You can learn and practice imagery from audio tapes or a book, but it's helpful to have a few sessions with an instructor to discover the techniques that work best for you.

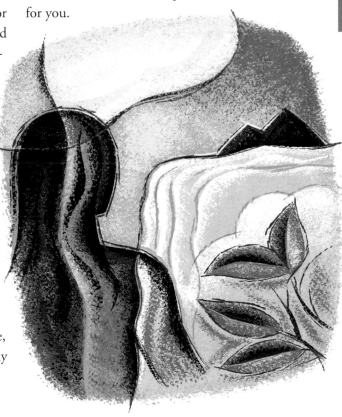

Sessions last from 30 to 60 minutes, and usually begin with a relaxation, meditation or breathing exercise. The instructor (or an audio tape) then guides you through a visualization exercise, encouraging you to chose specific images and sensations that have strong meaning for you. The type of exercise depends on your goal. To relieve anxiety, for example, you may want to revisit a scene when you were happy and safe. The smells, sounds, images and emotions of that time are uniquely yours: Recreating them in your imagination can recreate those same feelings of well-being in your body. To relieve pain, you might create a mental image of your symptoms and imagine them melting away, or being swept from your body. Another technique is to imagine yourself healthy and going about an activity you enjoy without pain or stress. Athletes have long used these techniques before a competition to visualize themselves performing perfectly. You can prepare yourself for a stressful upcoming event such as an uncomfortable medical procedure by imagining yourself sailing through the process successfully and easily.

Regular practice reinforces these positive feelings and their effect on your body and mind.

Scientific Evidence

Few studies look at visualization alone. Most have looked at imagery in combination

A Guided Imagery Exercise

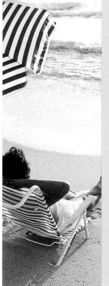

Imagine that you are at the ocean. … You are sitting comfortably on the beach under the shade of a large beach umbrella. … Feel the warm sand under you … and the warm, comfortable air around you … and the refreshing, soft breeze blowing through your hair. … Feel the warm moisture in the air upon your face. … Notice the smell of the ocean. … Imagine how beautiful, brilliantly blue the sky is….

You're sitting on the beach … feeling calm … peaceful … relaxed … comfortable…. You are watching the waves … as they grow and break … mesmerized as they go in and out from the shore…. You can hear the thundering of the waves as they break…. The only other sounds are those of the seagulls….

Notice how peaceful you feel … sitting on the beach … feeling in harmony with nature.

RESOURCES ✳ VISUALIZATION AND GUIDED IMAGERY

Organizations

Academy for Guided Imagery
P.O. Box 2070
Mill Valley, CA 94942
Phone: 800/726-2070
E-mail: strategicvisions@usa.net
Web site: http://www.healthy.net/agi
Has a referral list of practitioners and a catalogue of products.

Books

Creative Visualization, by Shakti Gawain. 1983. Bantam Books. Paperback. $6.50. Also available on audio tape.

Getting Well Again, by O. Carl Simonton, MD, Stephanie Matthews, James L. Creighton.
1992. Bantam. Paperback. $6.99.

Deep Healing: The Essence of Mind/Body Medicine, by Emmett Miller. 1997. Hay House. Paperback. $12.95. Also available on audio tape.

Audio Tapes

There are many imagery or visualization audio tapes. The best ones are those that work for you, so sample several. You can also make you own tapes of your favorite visualizations. See Using Mind–Body Audio Tapes, page 77.

with other mind–body techniques such as biofeedback and relaxation.

Many of the studies are flawed: A review of studies between 1982 and 1995 found studies have problems such as small size or lack of controls, but concluded there is still evidence that imagery and relaxation combinations can relieve pain (Wallace). However, a controlled study of the effects of relaxation and imagery on multiple sclerosis patients showed clinically significant reductions in anxiety (Maguire).

Visualization is used to support conventional medicine. O. Carl Simonton, MD, and colleagues created a stir in the 1970s when they announced patients taught to visualize an army of white cells gobbling up their cancer cells could extend their life span (Simonton). Other studies haven't confirmed that visualization extends life or cures disease (Spiegel 1). They have suggested, however, that visualization can improve immune function when combined with other relaxation techniques.

An uncontrolled study in Denmark gave 10 healthy people a one-hour relaxation and guided imagery session for 10 days, telling the people to imagine their immune systems getting stronger. They had a significant increase in natural killer cell function (Zachariae).

Expert Opinion

Visualization and guided imagery are variations on the same theme as meditation and biofeedback. They use quiet contemplation and focus, and can do much to relieve your pain and build a positive self-image. There are no side effects.

Finding a Practitioner

Visualization and guided imagery techniques are taught by a wide range of practitioners. Many mental health professionals use them, and they are used in stress reduction and relaxation programs. However, they are also offered by people who may not have any training. So be sure to check out the credentials of anyone you plan to consult.

Good Advice

• Be sure to focus on positive outcomes and situations. If someone suggests using visualization or imagery techniques to work out psychological issues or problems, be sure to consult a qualified mental health practitioner.

Costs

A session with a health professional is billed at regular rates ($40–$125) and may be covered by insurance, especially with your physician's prescription. Other rates vary widely.

HYPNOSIS

Hypnosis has been around for centuries and been used in many cultures to promote healing as well as for magic and religious trances. Modern hypnotism began in the 1770s when an Austrian doctor named Franz Anton Mesmer devised a theory of "animal magnetism" and began treating people with magnets. His magnet therapy was exposed as a fraud when his success turned out to be related to his ability to soothe and persuade people, or "mesmerize" them. Other doctors became interested in the medical uses of "mesmerism" to relieve pain, and later for psychotherapy.

Today hypnosis is an accepted medical treatment. But some may associate it with party stunts or villains who "put people into a trance" and make them do things against their will. Actually, hypnotism isn't "done" to you any more than meditation or visualization: It's yet another technique of altered consciousness to help focus attention and foster relaxation. It's estimated that between 5 percent and 30 percent of people are susceptible to hypnosis. You can learn to hypnotize yourself. In fact, some say all hypnosis is self-hypnosis.

When hypnotized, you enter into a restful state of very focused attention and acute awareness. You can concentrate intently, making it easier to use visualization, relaxation or other mind–body techniques. Hypnotism has long been used in psychotherapy and to reinforce changes in mental attitude or behavior, but it has been shown to be useful in other conditions as well. It is sometimes used, with varying success, to help people overcome addictions to smoking and alcohol. It can help people with arthritis and other painful conditions reduce and relieve pain, especially when used with other therapies.

What Happens in a Hypnosis Session

A hypnotherapy session is much like a guided imagery session. The practitioner guides you through a relaxation exercise, talking in a slow soothing voice. You may be led "deeper" into relaxation by being asked to count backwards, or to imagine walking up or down a long staircase. Once you are deeply relaxed, you will be aware of your surroundings but open to suggestions. The suggestions depend on the goals you have set for the session: You may work on relieving pain or planting positive ideas about your health.

The depth of your trance and the success of hypnotism for you depends on many things, including your willingness to be hypnotized and your imagination. Hypnotists say your subconscious mind won't accept unreasonable suggestions or go against your wishes. With practice, you can learn to invoke this deeply relaxed but aware state yourself. There are many books and tapes, but a session with a hypnotist can also teach these techniques.

Scientific Evidence

Hypnotism has a long history of therapeutic use, and studies show it can be effective for many disorders.

Studies have shown that it can relieve irritable bowel symptoms, sometimes completely (Harvey, Whorwell). It has also been used to treat fibromyalgia. In a randomized, controlled study of 40 people with hard-to-treat fibromyalgia,

the group assigned to hypnosis had a significantly greater decrease in pain, fatigue on awakening, and other symptoms than the group that had physical therapy (Haanen).

An uncontrolled study that looked at 19 people with arthritis pain found hypnotherapy decreased pain, anxiety and depression (Domangue). In a study of pain in cancer patients, hypnotism combined with a support group was shown to be more effective than the support group alone (Spiegel 2).

Expert Opinion

Hypnotism may help relieve pain, irritable bowel syndrome and other symptoms connected with arthritis. It's also an alternative to meditation, biofeedback and visualization. There is little risk of side effects.

Finding a Practitioner

Hypnotists are not regulated. Hypnosis is used by many mental health practitioners and a wide range of other practitioners. Several organization such as the National Guild of Hypnotists certify practitioners. It is also offered by people who may not have proper training. Be sure to check out the credentials of anyone you plan to consult.

Costs

A session with a health professional is billed at regular rates ($40–$125) and may be covered by your insurance. Other rates vary widely.

RESOURCES ✳ HYPNOSIS

Organizations
National Guild of Hypnotists
P.O. Box 308
Merrimack, NH 03054-0308
Phone: 603/429-9438
E-mail: ngh@ngh.net
Web site: http://www.ngh.net
Represents 7,000 hypnotists worldwide.
Has information and a referral list.

American Council of Hypnotist
Examiners (ACHE)
700 South Central Avenue
Glendale, CA 91204-2011
Phone: 818/242-1159
Provides a referral list of hypnotists
certified by ACHE. It does not require
licensing in a health or mental health
profession.

Using Mind-Body Audio Tapes

Many relaxation, guided meditation and visualization audio tapes are available for home use. These can be very useful in guiding you to a state of peace and relaxation, and regular use can help you break cycles of pain and tension.

Choosing a tape depends on personal preference. Look for tapes produced by or endorsed by a health organization or well-known practitioners (see Resources). However, the best tape is the one that works for you. Some techniques will be more appealing and easier for you to practice. Also, you may find you respond to some voices more than others, or may prefer music with the instructions. Listen to several to see which you like, or make your own by recording an exercise you like.

- Choose tapes with specific verbal directions to guide you through the practice, rather than music-only tapes.

- Find a quiet place where you won't be disturbed while the tape plays. Be sure you are warm enough and comfortable so you can relax and remain still.

- Try to use the tape at the same time every day to set up a habit of relaxation.

- Don't worry if you fall asleep before the tape is over. But don't use the tape at bedtime as a sleep aid: The goal is to learn to relax while you are awake.

- To get the best results, use the tape daily for several weeks until you have learned the "relaxation response." Eventually, you'll be able to use the technique without listening to the instructions, but you may want to use the tape at times when you feel especially stressed to help you relax and focus.

RELAXATION TECHNIQUES:
WORKING WITH TENSION AND BREATH

Before we can begin to relax, we have to learn how to recognize tension. Many of us just don't know how much tension we are carrying, because we've being doing it for so long it feels "normal." You can learn to release tension by practicing muscle relaxation and breathing exercises. The three techniques described here are at the core of most stress reduction programs, and are often combined with other therapies. They are very powerful, easy to learn and can be practiced at home.

RESOURCES *
RELAXATION TECHNIQUES

Book
The Breathing Book: Vitality and Good Health Through Essential Breath Work, by Donna Farhi. 1996. Henry Holt and Company. Paperback. $17.95.

Audio Tape
Guided Body Scan Meditation and Yoga 1.
Available by writing Stress Reduction Tapes, P.O. Box 547, Lexington, MA 02173. Add $1 handing charge. Or order through http://www.mindfulnesstapes.com

Breathing Lessons

Everybody has to breathe to stay alive so there's no need for breathing lessons, right? Wrong.

Research and observation show what Eastern health systems have long known: that the way we breathe reflects and affects what's going on in our mind and body. You've seen it yourself. Powerful negative emotions such as pain, anger or fear are expressed in short, shallow, quick breaths – or can even cause you to hold your breath. Powerful positive emotions such as pleasure, love and deep relaxation are reflected in long, deep, nourishing breathing.

By learning techniques to control your breathing, you can better cope with stress, pain and negative emotions. Breathing techniques are a key part of many relaxation and stress reduction courses. Deep breathing is also taught in yoga, tai chi and qi gong (see Moving Medicine, page 97). Lamaze childbirth exercises are based on breathing techniques, and athletes use conscious breathing to improve performance. You can use steady, deep breathing to turn off the fight-or-flight response, lower blood pressure, ease panic attacks and control pain. Other techniques can show you how to use your breath to energize yourself.

How to Practice Full-Body Breathing

Here's a basic breathing exercise to make you aware of how you are breathing and show you how to practice abdominal (or full-body) breathing for relaxation.

Find a quiet place where you won't be disturbed. Loosen any tight clothing and take off your shoes. Lie down if you can. If not, find a sitting posture that's comfortable.

Put one hand on your stomach just below your breastbone and take a few deep breaths. Notice if your hand moves when you breathe. Most of us only use our upper chest for breathing. Take a few more breaths, breathing in and out through your nose, allowing your stomach and ribcage to expand under your hand as you breathe.

Next, put your hand on your abdomen below your waist, and notice if it moves. Take a few more deep breaths, filling up your abdomen, your ribcage and your chest. Let the breath out slowly. It may help to count slowly to three on each in breath and again on each out breath. You may be overcome with the urge to yawn: Let it happen.

After a few minutes, allow your breathing to return to normal. Don't keep taking deep, big breaths, or you'll make yourself dizzy. Just breath in and out normally, but focus on bringing the breathing all the way down into your abdomen so that you breathe in and out with your entire body. It's easier to practice abdominal breathing if you are lying down. You can place a book on your stomach or abdomen, and expand your breathing to make the book rise and fall. If you feel dizzy or lightheaded, stop and return to your normal breathing until the feeling passes.

Continue full-body breathing for five to 10 breaths. Allow your body to relax with each out breath, letting it sink down into the floor or chair. You can use visualization to help you relax even more. Imagine that you are breathing in light and breathing out pain, or that you are melting into the floor below you. As you come to the end of the practice, take a deep cleansing breath. You may be a bit light-headed when you finish, so move carefully at first.

You can practice this breathing exercise in a shorter version whenever you feel stressed. Sometimes just three or four full-body breaths can center you. Many find this also helps them overcome urges for tobacco and other addictive substances.

Untying Your Muscles and Mind

The following exercises teach you how to recognize and release tension. In the progressive muscle relaxation exercise, you methodically tense and relax parts of your body, muscle by muscle, noticing the difference between tension and relaxation. With the body scan exercise, you bring attention to your body section by section, just noticing and accepting the way you feel. These exercises also utilize breathing lessons and visualization (see page 79) to help you relax and tune in to your body.

How to Practice Progressive Muscle Relaxation

Find a quiet place to lie down where you won't be disturbed for 15 to 20 minutes. Get comfortable, supporting any body parts that are achy or tender: You may want to put a pillow under your knees and neck. If pain is overwhelming any part of your body as you do this exercise, be very gentle tensing muscles in that area. It may be enough just to bring awareness to the tension or pain with an in breath, and then exhale and imagine it letting go.

Take a few deep cleansing breaths and allow your body to feel the floor or mat beneath you. Bring your attention to your right foot. Inhale and tense the muscles of your foot and calf, hold for three or four seconds, then exhale and release all the tension at once, letting the foot flop down. Working your way up the leg, tense and release your knee and thigh. Repeat on the left leg. Moving to your torso, tense and relax the buttocks, then stomach and chest. Bring your attention to your hands and arms, starting with your fingers, and tense and release each section. Now move your shoulders up tight around your ears, tense and release. Scrunch up your face, hold, and release. Open your eyes and mouth as wide as you can, stick out your tongue, and release. Finally, tense every muscle that you can, hold for a few seconds, and then let everything drop into relaxation.

Repeat the full-body scrunch two times. Relax into the mat and feel everything letting go and melting away. Lie quietly for a few minutes, or use this relaxed state as an entry to move into a breathing exercise, meditation or visualization.

Scientific Evidence

Good evidence is readily available that relaxation techniques, usually used in combination, can ease pain, depression and anxiety. The relaxation therapies described here are often part of stress reduction programs, or are used with other practices. (See Scientific Evidence for biofeedback and meditation.)

A randomized, controlled trial looked at the effects of a combination of psychological therapies on rheumatoid arthritis patients and found significant reduction in pain, disease activity and anxiety. Researchers thought relaxation training may have been the important component of the program (Bradley).

A group of eight people with irritable bowel syndrome received an eight-week series of classes in progressive muscle relaxation, and practiced regularly at home. Another group of eight received no relaxation training. The relaxation group showed significantly more improvement than the control group (Blanchard).

Several studies show children respond well to relaxation techniques. A controlled study of 40 children and teens hospitalized with adjustment disorder and depression looked at the effects of a one-hour class that included yoga, a brief massage and progressive muscle relaxation. There was a decrease both in self-reported anxiety and fidgeting as well as a decrease in the stress hormone cortisol in the relaxation group, while no changes were noted in the control group, which watched a one-hour relaxing videotape (Platania-Solazzo).

An uncontrolled study looked at 13 children between the ages of 4 and 16 who had juvenile rheumatoid arthritis. In eight individual sessions they were taught progressive muscle relaxation, guided imagery and meditative breathing. Their pain reduced substantially, and that relief continued at six- and 12-month follow-ups (Walco 1). The same researcher found children with juvenile primary fibromyalgia had similar results from progressive muscle relaxation (Walco 2).

Expert Opinion

These techniques have good evidence to show they can help with chronic pain, stress and depression. You may think you don't want to increase your body awareness, at least of painful areas. With these techniques, however, you may gain an awareness of how and where you hold tension and pain and how to relieve it. They are well worth trying.

Finding a Practitioner

Many physical therapists, yoga instructors and mental health practitioners use these and other techniques to help you learn how to unknot muscles and relax a tense mind and body, or to energize you. Look for these in a stress reduction course through your local hospital or health organization. You can also learn many variations of these exercises from audio tapes, videos and books. Some people make

How to Practice a Body Scan

In this exercise, you learn to relax tension and relieve pain by becoming aware of and accepting your body just as it is, in this moment. That's a difficult task for some of us, especially when our bodies are the cause of pain and discomfort. The exercise described here can help. It's adapted from a mindfulness-based stress reduction practice developed by Jon Kabat-Zinn, PhD, at the University of Massachusetts Medical Center.

It's important to do this exercise every day for at least two weeks, to create a habit of relaxation. It will take about 45 minutes. That may seem like a big time commitment, but it is time you spend relaxing and caring for your mind and body.

The description here will give you an idea of the exercise, but it's best to do this with an audio tape, as your attention can wander and the voice on the tape brings you back to the practice. Don't worry if you fall asleep during the exercise: That's a sign you are relaxing, but don't use this technique to fall asleep.

Find a quiet place to lie down where you won't be disturbed and make yourself as comfortable as possible. You may want to cover yourself with a blanket to stay warm as you relax. Close your eyes and take a few full-body breaths, feeling the breath move in and out through your body. Feel the way your body settles into the mat or floor.

Bring your attention to the toes of your right foot. See if you can direct your breathing to your toes, so that it feels as if you are breathing into your toes and out from your toes. Allow yourself to feel any sensation from your toes – or lack of sensation – without doing anything. Just breathe and observe.

When you are ready to move on, take a deep breath all the way down to your toes, and allow your toes to "dissolve" as you exhale. Then move your attention to the sole of your foot, the top of the foot, the ankle, and so on throughout your body. Repeat the breathing and bring full attention to each part of your body, observing sensations without judgment and letting go of each section as you move on. If your mind wanders away, gently bring it back to the breath and to the body section you were working with when your attention strayed.

If pain intrudes or overwhelms you, you might find it difficult to keep your attention on that specific part of your body. If this happens, don't worry. Stay with an awareness of that region as long as you feel you can (even one minute is good) and then see if you can let go, and move on to focus on another part of the body. If you have a great deal of pain, it will help you to learn this and other techniques from an instructor (see Resources). Eventually you will be able to move your attention with greater confidence through the painful areas, experiencing the sensations as they are and letting go of them as you move on to the next part of your body.

Don't hurry through this exercise. The process is the point. When you have come to the end, give yourself a few minutes to experience the deep relaxation before getting up.

their own audio tapes, or have a loved one make one, by reading and recording exercises available in many books.

Cautions

! Tensing muscles that haven't been used much may bring on cramps or pain at first. If you have severe rheumatoid arthritis, fibromyalgia or are having a flare, start progressive muscle relaxation gently. Tighten your muscles just enough to be aware of the tension: Awareness is the important point, not how hard you squeeze your muscles.

! Breathing exercises may make you lightheaded until you get the hang of it, and deep relaxation may also make you a bit wobbly at first. So take a minute when you finish the exercises to reorient yourself. Get up slowly, being careful to check your balance.

Good Advice

• Bringing attention to your body may increase your awareness of pain at first. This is normal. However, the pain should fade as you begin to relax. If the awareness of pain continues to override any relaxation sensations, consult a practitioner. There are a number of techniques, and one may be more effective than another for you.

Costs

You may find these practices included in other therapies, such as biofeedback, yoga or

Group Therapy and Support Groups

Support groups and group therapy have been a great help to many with chronic illnesses. A group of fibromyalgia patients also improved after a six-month group therapy program that emphasized mind–body techniques, coping strategies and support sessions of significant others (Bennett).

Your doctor or treatment team may be able to direct you to a local group. If that doesn't get you what you want, try these options:

- Call one of the national organizations listed, such as the Arthritis Foundation, and ask about local groups or contacts for organizations that represent specific kinds of arthritis.

- Ask your doctor who to contact at a local hospital or medical center.

- Ask at your church, synagogue or other religious center.

meditation; or they may be taught in a stress reduction program. Rates vary widely: Meditation may be free of charge, yoga classes range from about $4 to $20 per session. Stress reduction program costs vary but generally run from around $150 to $700 for a six- or eight-week session that meets once a week. A session with a health professional is billed at regular rates ($40–$125) and may be covered by insurance.

STRESS REDUCTION AND RELAXATION PROGRAMS

These programs combine many of the therapies discussed in this chapter, often along with yoga. They are often offered in classes that meet once a week for six to eight weeks through patient-education courses at hospitals, at chronic pain centers, and by some businesses and corporations as an employee benefit.

The benefits of stress reduction have been well-documented, and a growing number of medical professionals consider these programs beneficial for almost any kind of chronic illness. The techniques can significantly reduce pain, relieve depression and generally improve quality of life for many, and there are virtually no side effects or risks. These are intended to complement conventional medical treatment, not replace it. But people who use these techniques may be able to reduce their reliance on pain medication or other drugs.

Stress reduction programs have been shown to work for people of all ages and from any walk of life – including those who never thought they could be doing something as far out as meditating. Participating with others in a group process that spans several months may also benefit those who have been isolated in their pain or disability. For an idea of how a program is conducted, see Part III, "Healing from Within" of the PBS video by Bill Moyers called "Healing and the Mind" (available at many public libraries).

Scientific Evidence

Stress management programs have had good results for chronic pain management (Kabat-Zinn 3), and for helping people with many symptoms related to arthritis.

In a randomized, controlled trial, 37 people with psoriasis undergoing ultraviolet light therapy were divided into two groups. One group participated in mindfulness meditation along with the light therapy; the other group received only the light therapy. Those who had the stress reduction therapy were able to clear their skin lesions significantly faster than the control group (Kabat-Zinn 4).

A randomized, controlled trial of people with irritable bowel syndrome compared a six-session stress management program with conventional treatment. Two-thirds of those who learned relaxation and other techniques had fewer attacks of less severity, and the relief lasted for at least a year after the program. Few of those on conventional therapy had any benefit (Shaw).

A group of people with fibromyalgia met weekly for six months for a program that

Organizations

The Mind–Body Medical Institute
Division of Behavioral Medicine
New England Deaconess Hospital
One Deaconess Road
Boston, MA 02215
Phone: 617/632-9525
E-mail: mbmi@caregroup.harvard.edu
Web site: http://www.mindbody.harvard.edu
Has information about mind–body programs for different medical conditions, as well as referral to a program near you.

Stress Reduction Clinic
Center for Mindfulness in Medicine, Health Care and Society
University of Massachusetts Medical Center
Worcester, MA 01655
Phone: 508/856-2656
For information about mindfulness and stress reduction as well as referral to a program near you.

Book

Wherever You Go, There You Are, by Jon Kabat-Zinn. 1994. New York. Hyperion. Paperback. $13.95.

included behavioral modification therapy, stress reduction and exercise. The control group showed no significant improvement, whereas 70 percent of the therapy group had a 25 percent improvement in tender points and overall disease impact. Participants continued to show improvement two years after the program ended (Bennett).

A randomized, controlled trial tested the effects of stress management training on people with rheumatoid arthritis. The stress management group showed statistically significant improvement in helplessness, coping, pain and health status (Parker 2).

Expert Opinion

Reducing stress and pain without medications can help many with arthritis and related disorders. The techniques do require a personal commitment: They must be practiced regularly to work, and that's not easy for some. But those who finish a program show long-term benefits even if they stop practicing. These programs are well worth the investment of time and money.

Finding a Program

Contact the resources on page 86 for a referral to a stress reduction program. You can also ask your doctor, a local health maintenance organization or inquire at an area hospital or university.

Cautions

! Before enrolling in a stress reduction program, check out its background and the credentials of the practitioner. It's best to pick a program affiliated with a health facility you know or with a nationally known organization.

Good Advice

• To be effective, these programs take time: both to go to sessions, and to do the daily practice. If you decide to enroll in a program, make it a priority. Tell yourself that you are doing this for your health.

Costs

Program costs vary but generally run from around $150 to $700 for a six- or eight-week session that meets once a week. Your insurance may cover all or part of the fee. They are also offered at a discount through a growing number of health maintenance organizations and community health education programs.

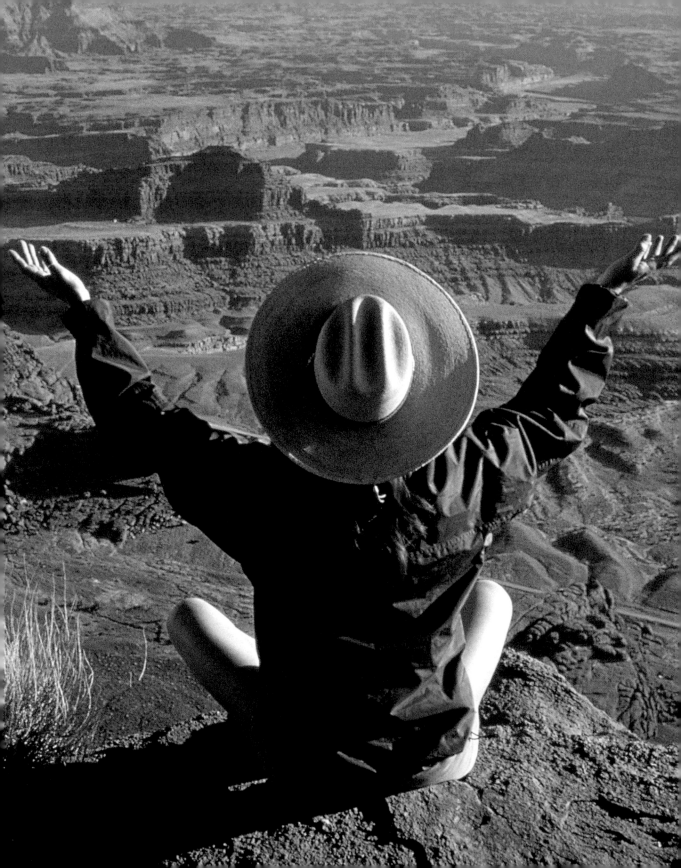

Prayer and Spirituality

THE ROLE OF FAITH

Americans are a spiritual people. According to Gallup polls, 95 percent of us believe in God or a universal spirit, and 76 percent of us pray on a regular basis. Moreover, 79 percent of Americans believe that faith helps people recover from illness. It is generally accepted that prayer and other spiritual practices can help us cope with suffering, offer comfort in times of illness and depression, and perhaps even help in healing.

Many people with arthritis and related musculoskeletal disorders think so. Several studies show that prayer is one of the most commonly used "alternative" therapies for arthritis – and often rated one of the most helpful (Bill-Harvey, Pioro-Boisset). Yet health professionals barely ever mention religion and spirituality in connection with health. One study that reviewed more than 1,000 articles in seven major medical journals found only 12 contained references to spiritual or religious practices (Orr).

It wasn't always this way. Historically, religion and medicine have been intertwined. In many cultures, the healer was also a priest or priestess, and monasteries and convents were the earliest hospitals. Many religious organizations still operate hospitals and health centers today. About 300 years ago, the scientific revolution separated the practice of medicine from religion. Today, medicine is taking another look at the role of faith and spiritual practice. Research in behavioral medicine has shown that the powerful interactions of mind, body and spirit can have profound effects on our health. Prayer and spirituality may play important roles as well.

There are many kinds of prayer and spiritual practices, but in general they share a belief or faith in higher powers. The terms religion and spirituality are often used interchangeably, but they have different meanings. Religion refers to an organization or institution with established rituals, beliefs and practices and a community of others who share the same beliefs. It's expressed by attending services or other meetings of the religious organization. Spirituality, on the other hand, is a personal search for meaning and connection with a higher power. Spirituality is part of religion, but a person can be spiritual without belonging to a religion or attending religious services.

Scientific Evidence

It's difficult to study the effects of prayer and faith on health. Studies that look at the role of prayer and faith tend to look at those who practice a religion. There's a practical reason for this: It's easier to design a study that looks at actions, such as attending services, than a study that looks at inner intent. Many studies tend to show positive effects of religion, suggesting that those who attend services have better health. These studies, however, are often criticized for being poorly done.

Nourishing the Soul

Here are some spiritual practices that bring many comfort and serenity.

- Pray or meditate every day. A short period of daily prayer or meditation can help us find peace in a hectic world, and the deep rest that can come with this practice is powerful medicine. Studies do show meditation can relieve stress and ease chronic pain. See Meditation, page 62.

- Find a spiritual group. It might be worthwhile to explore a spiritual practice with a community of others who share your values. You might want to visit different kinds of services and spiritual meetings to find one that suits you. But don't "church hop" too long before settling on one or you'll miss one of the proven benefits of a spiritual practice: the companionship and support that comes from being a member of a community.

- Attend services regularly. Solitary spiritual practice may appeal to you, but studies suggest that it is the regular attendance at services that is good for your health. Attending services makes you part of a community and gives you social, moral and physical support when you need help or are ill.

- Make a retreat. A retreat from the world to a spiritual center nourishes your soul. It can help you relieve stress and reorganize your priorities. Many religious and spiritual organizations offer weekend or even one-day retreats to refresh and renew yourself.

Some of the effects on health suggested by studies of religion include:

- Better health practices. Several studies show people who attend religious services take better care of their health. A study that looked at 5,286 people over 28 years showed frequent attenders not only had lower mortality rates, but also were more likely to stop smoking, increase exercising, increase social contacts and stay married (Strawbridge).

- Longer life. In a five-year study of 1,931 elderly people, those who attended religious services had a 24 percent lower mortality rate than those who did not, even after adjusting for variables such as chronic disease or smoking (Oman).

- Better recovery after serious surgery. People

Organizations

There are many organizations specific to religious denominations or practices. The ones listed here are of general interest.

National Institute for Healthcare Research
6110 Executive Boulevard, Suite 908
Rockville, MD 20852
Phone: 301/984-7162
E-mail: nihr@nihr.org
Web site:
http://www.nihr.org/clinical/prg_cal.html
NIHR conducts and produces reports on scientific research on the relationship between spirituality and physical, mental and social health.

The Park Ridge Center for the Study of Health, Faith and Ethics
211 E. Ontario, Suite 800
Chicago, IL 60611-3215
Phone: 312/266-2222
Web site: http://www.prchfe.org
The Park Center Bulletin is on the Web site, and offered free of charge.

The John Templeton Foundation
E-mail: info@templeton.org
Web site: http://www.templeton.org
A non-profit organization that studies the role of spirituality and morality.

Trinity Church Institute for Christian Renewal
New Creation Healing Center
148 Plaistrow Road
Plaistrow, NH 03865
Phone: 603/382-0273

Books

The Faith Factor: Proof of the Healing Power of Prayer, by Dale A. Matthews and Connie Clark. 1999. New York. Viking-Penguin. Paperback. $13.95.

Healing Words: The Power of Prayer and the Practice of Medicine, by Larry Dossey, MD. 1993. New York. Harper Collins. Paperback. $6.50.

The Heart of Buddha's Teaching: Transforming Suffering into Peace, Joy, and Liberation, by Thich Nhat Hanh. Parallax Press. Hardcover. $22.50.

The Heart's Code: Tapping the Wisdom and Power of Our Heart Energy, by Paul Pearsall. 1999. Broadway Books. Paperback. $13.

The Miracle of Mindfulness: A Manual on Meditation, by Thich Nhat Hahn. 1988. Boston, MA. Beacon Press. Paperback. $12.

Prayer Is Good Medicine: How to Reap the Healing Benefits of Prayer, by Larry Dossey, MD. 1997. Harper Collins. Paperback. $12.

Timeless Healing: The Power and Biology of Belief, by Herbert Benson, MD. 1997. Fireside. Paperback. $14.

Web Sites

First Church of Cyberspace
This ecumenical Web site features information on many topics related to religion, including links to other sites.
http://www.godweb.org

Spirituality and Health
Sponsored by the Trinity Church, Wall Street, this site has articles on spirituality, prayer and religion, movie and book reviews, and interactive articles.
http://www.spiritualityhealth.com/about/abus.html

with a social support group and religious faith were three times more likely to be alive six months after open-heart surgery than those who were not religious (Oxman).

- Less use of medical services. People who attended church weekly or more often were significantly less likely to have been admitted to a hospital and spent fewer days in the hospital than those who attended church less often (Koenig 1).

- Faster recovery from depression. Among depressed older people who were hospitalized, those with a religious faith recovered from depression faster (Koenig 2).

Other studies – also with mixed results – have looked at the effects of intercessory prayer, where people pray on behalf of another. Those who are praying may never have met the people who are being prayed for, who may be physically distant and not even know they are the subject of prayers.

One uncontrolled study looked at the effects of two kinds of prayer on 40 patients with moderately severe rheumatoid arthritis. All participants received a three-day in-person prayer treatment that included six hours of education and six hours of "laying on of hands" over the affected joints. Half of the group received an additional six months of distant prayer from individuals in other cities. All participants received conventional treatments, and there was no control group of people who received neither a prayer nor

education intervention. One year later, there were significant clinical improvements for the group as a whole, including a statistically significant reduction in the number of tender and swollen joints and in the level of disability and pain. Those who received distant prayer did not show any additional improvement (Matthews).

An often-quoted study of coronary patients who were prayed for by a Christian group found they had fewer complications than those not prayed for (Byrd). Neither doctors, patients, nor those praying knew who was being prayed for. This study has been criticized for its methodology, but created interest in further research.

A more recent study looked at AIDS patients receiving intercessory, distant prayer for 10 weeks (Sicher). They had less severe illness, fewer new AIDS-related illnesses, and had significantly fewer doctors' visits than the group not prayed for. However, their CD4 counts, a standard measure of AIDS progress, weren't different from the control group.

Critics say many of the studies that show positive health effects from religion are flawed, use poor methods or don't take many variables into account. A review of more than a dozen studies found the connection between religion and health to be weak and inconsistent, even in the best-done studies (Sloan). For example, a study that showed church attendance is connected with better health didn't consider that people who can go to church are healthier to begin with. People with poorer health are less likely to be able to go to services.

There is good evidence that meditation – which can be a form of prayer – can relieve pain, depression and anxiety (see Meditation page 62). There is also some mixed evidence for the effectiveness of therapeutic touch (page 126) and reiki (page 126), in which a practitioner channels universal energy into those who need healing.

However, critics say positive results for prayer may reflect a placebo effect: People with religious faith expect to be sick less, and so they are. Also, many of the studies might really show the value of companionship and community, not religion. Interestingly, these two criticisms seem to reinforce the value of a religious practice, because faith and companionship are key parts of most religions.

Some critics have an ethical concern that linking health with spirituality could do harm. There are some false ideas that illness is a punishment for sins or the result of a lack of faith. It's possible some will connect illness with moral failure or weakness, and health with "goodness." This could add a burden of guilt or blame to those already struggling with a chronic illness (Sloan).

Expert Opinion

There is strong scientific evidence to suggest that praying or other spiritual practices will improve your health. If your health does improve, the exact role of religious faith can't be separated from the good effects of social support and positive attitudes that come along with most religions or spiritual groups.

People have been finding comfort, meaning and inspiration from prayer and other spiritual practices for thousands of years. It could be that adding or deepening the spiritual aspects in your life could be good for you and your arthritis. Your arthritis may not improve if you pray or attend services, but the process may make you feel better and help you cope better with the symptoms of arthritis.

Cautions

! Don't expect spiritual practice to "cure" you, or feel you have failed if it seems that your prayers are not answered. Many of the rewards of a spiritual practice come from the process, and are not aimed at results.

! Beware of those who promise that following their faith will cure your arthritis, or who ask for a large sums of money. Responsible spiritual leaders are concerned with your spiritual health and healing. They don't promise cures for physical ailments, or charge for their services. Don't sign your savings over to any organization without first getting legal or financial advice from an expert not connected to that organization.

Good Advice

- Those who follow a specific path may believe theirs is the only or best path and may condemn other religions or practices. However, that may not be the path for you.
- Trust your feelings. A spiritual search is a personal journey. It's your body and your faith.

Costs

Spirituality and prayer are free of charge. Many religious organizations ask for donations to join and for offerings at services or meetings. However, these are not large amounts and no truly spiritual organization turns away those who can't afford to pay.

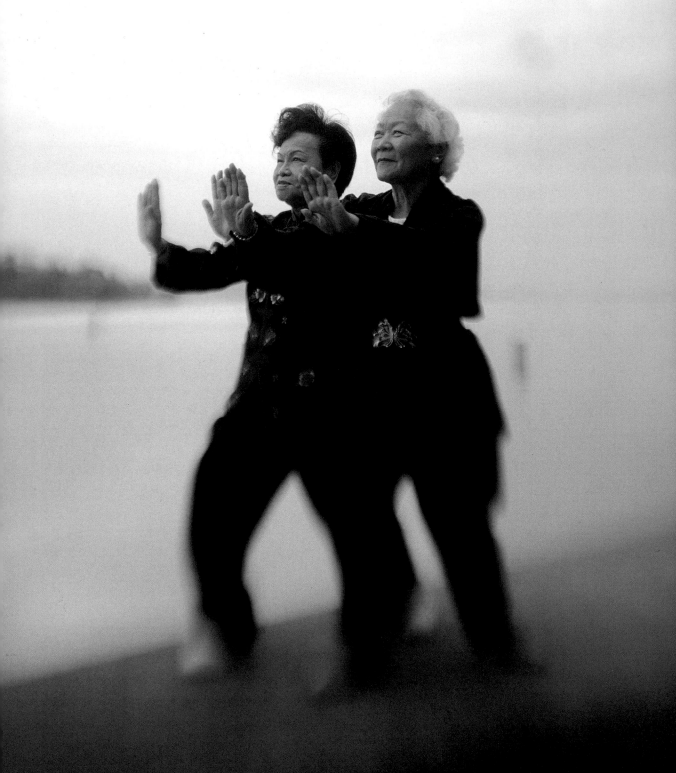

Moving Medicine

GENTLE EXERCISE
ALTERNATIVES

You know you should exercise more: Study after study confirms that those who exercise stay healthier, live longer and cope better with chronic pain. And you don't have to be told again that it's even more important for people with arthritis and related diseases to keep those joints and muscles moving.

But it isn't easy to work out when a short session at the gym leaves you aching – or when even everyday activities hurt so much the very thought of exercise makes you wince.

The therapies in this chapter may get you moving again. They exercise the body, mind and

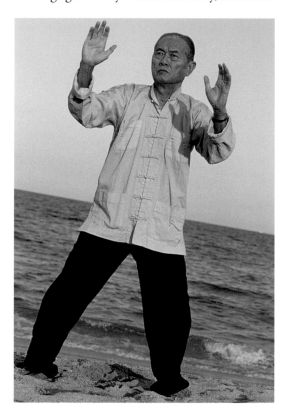

spirit, and may help improve the quality of your life. Unlike exercise programs with a "no pain, no gain" philosophy, these systems encourage you to move within your limits. They help you learn how best to use your unique body while increasing your levels of fitness and flexibility.

Three disciplines from the ancient East – yoga, tai chi chuan and qi gong – offer alternatives to joint-jarring, muscle-straining exercise, yet give many of the benefits of an athletic workout. They strengthen muscles and improve balance, which helps relieve stress on tender joints; increase circulation to joints and muscles; and promote the release of endorphins, the body's "feel-good" chemicals that relieve stress and depression.

Three 20th-century movement education programs – the Alexander technique, Feldenkrais method and Trager approach – were developed to improve ease of movement. They can help you learn to correct movement habits that contribute to pain, and teach you to move more easily.

These techniques have mental and spiritual benefits as well. Because they focus on mental and physical relaxation, deep breathing, and developing body awareness, they can give some of the proven benefits of meditation and deep relaxation as well as those of exercise. Those who practice faithfully often say their improved mobility reduces their need for pain-killing drugs.

These programs work at any level of fitness. Each is used by actors, dancers and elite athletes as well as people with many ailments, including osteoarthritis, rheumatoid arthritis, fibromyalgia, and other joint or muscle problems. They can be modified to be done from a bed or a wheelchair, and have been used to help people learn to move correctly after joint replacement surgery.

None of these requires any special clothing or equipment, and after you've learned the basics they can be done just about anywhere.

Doctors and physical therapists who know about these methods often recommend them or use some of the techniques in their practice. In fact, some have become so mainstream you may find them at your local hospital, community center or health club.

But they don't do everything: They don't give an aerobic workout or all of the benefits of weight lifting. As you use them to build up strength and energy, you may want to combine them with exercise such as walking, non-impact aerobics (where the foot never completely leaves the floor), water aerobics, weight training, or riding a recumbent stationary bike.

Cautions

Before you begin: Ask your doctor or physical therapist about any general cautions or specific movements you should *not* do. Those with osteoarthritis in the neck should not do certain yoga postures such as the headstand, for example.

❗ Don't eat heavily or drink alcohol for at least two hours before practice.

❗ Be gentle with a joint that is inflamed (swollen, red, hot), putting it only through its range of motion. Modify your workout when you are having a flare or feel fatigued.

❗ If you are taking glucocorticoids, take special care. Long-term steroid use can leave your bones fragile.

❗ If you are taking painkillers, be aware they may mask pain. Without pain to warn you, you may go beyond your limits.

❗ Do not exercise too close to bedtime. Although gentle, these exercises energize body and mind, and may keep you awake.

Good Advice

• Be sure to seek a qualified instructor, and be sure he or she has experience working with your condition. If you have severe joint or muscle disease, you may want to choose a practitioner who is also a physical therapist or who works closely with one.

• Warm stiff joints and muscles before exercising: A warm bath or shower before class may make moving easier.

• Never push yourself or let an instructor push you beyond your limits, and don't do anything that hurts or adds to your existing pain. These are not competitive exercises. If a movement hurts, stop immediately and work with your instructor to modify it.

• Trust your instincts. Are you comfortable with the instructor? Does this practice make you feel better? Do you enjoy it? If not, stop and try something else.

YOGA

Yoga is an ancient system of mental, physical and spiritual training practiced daily by millions of people of all ages and all levels of wellness. A philosophy and devotional practice, it is part of the traditional Indian holistic healing system called Ayurveda (see page 29). For thousands of years, it has been used as a way to bring the body, mind and spirit into harmony. In fact, the very word "yoga" means union.

There are several branches of yoga practice, including a devotional form called bhakti yoga and the meditation of raja yoga. Most Westerners know the form called hatha yoga, a system of gentle stretches and balancing exercises that balance energy and provide low-impact, full-body conditioning.

Daily yoga practice can improve flexibility, increase muscle strength and help you relax. Yoga practitioners claim these exercises also maintain health and can help myriad ailments, including depression and chronic pain. They increase circulation, lower cholesterol, and are said to balance the immune and hormonal systems.

There are several schools of hatha yoga, which can range from a slow-motion meditation to a vigorous workout. All are centered around a series of carefully crafted postures, called asanas; and breathing techniques, called pranayama. The postures include sitting, standing and prone poses, performed with full concentration and careful attention to breathing and sensations in your body.

Don't try to learn yoga from a book or a video. It's important to study with an instructor who has been trained and certified by a yoga school, and who has experience teaching people with your type of arthritis. Look for a beginners' class, or a class for senior citizens where the pace is slow and where the teacher modifies the postures to match the ability of each student.

After you've learned the basics, you can practice along with a video or audio tape. However, it's a good idea to go to classes every so often, to be sure you are doing the postures correctly.

What Happens in a Yoga Class

Don't be intimidated by yoga videos that feature sleek bodies performing demanding poses. A beginners' yoga class typically is composed of people of all ages and stages of fitness, flexibility and flab, most often wearing loose-fitting tops and sweatpants. The postures are done barefoot on a non-slip mat or rug.

Sessions usually begin with deep breathing exercises and some gentle overall stretches. You'll be encouraged to move at your own pace, never pushing. A good instructor will help you modify postures, or offer props such as rolled towels or pillows.

The teacher demonstrates each posture, and then directs the class, checking that each student is performing it correctly and without straining. A few may be able to imitate the instructor's postures, while others may only be able to move a fraction of the distance. That's fine. The benefits of yoga come from working with your body within your abilities, and not from striving for an ideal pose. Only move as far into the pose as is comfortable for you.

Full-body breathing is an important part of yoga. As you perform the poses, you will notice that breathing and stretching open your chest and promote relaxation. Special yogic breathing exercises called pranayama can soothe or energize the body and mind. Standing poses will help your balance and increase your lower body strength. Poses performed sitting or lying on your back or stomach build muscle strength and flexibility.

Classes usually end with a brief meditation or deep relaxation exercise. Many find yoga does promote a union of body, mind and spirit, leaving them energized and peaceful.

Classes typically last from an hour to 90 minutes. A weekly yoga class will help you make sure you are doing the poses properly. But it's important to practice yoga more often: Daily practice is recommended. A basic routine can take 15 minutes to an hour, depending on the time you have and how much you need to unwind.

You may prefer to practice a few minutes of yoga first thing in the morning, to prepare for the day. Others prefer to do yoga at mid-day to relax and re-energize for the afternoon, or in the early evening to unwind from stress. However, avoid doing yoga – or any exercise – right before bedtime or after eating.

Scientific Evidence

There are many claims and case studies about the health benefits for yoga, but most of the studies are poorly done or lack controls. Still, they suggest regular yoga practice can relieve anxiety better than diazepan (Sahasi), reduce depression (Khumar), and increase alertness and well-being.

One study that compares yoga to relaxation and visualization found that pranayama (yogic breathing) produced a significantly greater feeling of alertness than the other techniques, and that a daily 30-minute program of breathing exercises and asanas had a "marked invigorating" effect on mood and physical energy (Wood).

A 1998 randomized, single-blind controlled trial looked at the effect of yoga on 42 people with carpal tunnel syndrome. Half of the people practiced yoga, and half wore wrist splints. At the end of eight weeks, the yoga group had significant improvement in grip strength and pain reduction (Garfinkel 1).

Sample Asanas

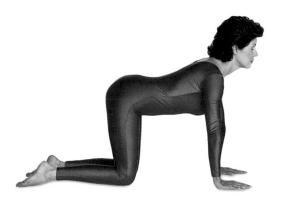

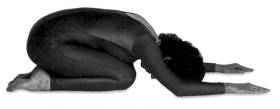

CHILD'S POSE

A relaxation posture that comforts and relaxes your body.

CAT

The cat pose stretches and strengthens the muscles of the low back.

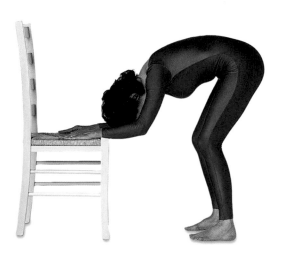

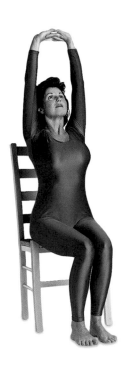

STANDING FORWARD BEND

Forward bending postures help keep the spine flexible. The pose is shown here modified with a chair.

ARM STRETCH

This stretch opens up the rib cage and promotes shoulder range of motion.

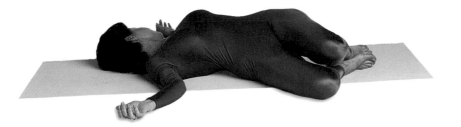

LYING SPINAL TWIST

Spinal twists help maintain side-to-side
mobility.

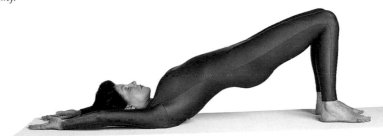

BRIDGE

The bridge is a backward bend. It is
performed to complement and balance
the forward bending postures.

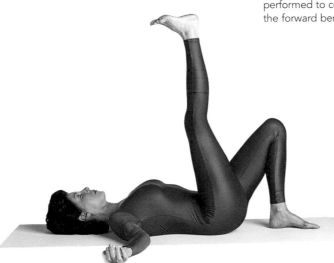

SINGLE LEG RAISE

Leg raises can be done with one leg
bent, or with both legs straight. They
strengthen the muscles of the low
back and abdomen.

RESOURCES * YOGA

Organizations

The American Yoga Association
P.O. Box 19986
Sarasota, FL 34276
Phone: 800/226-5859 or 941/927-4977
See Web site at right.

Yoga Research Center
P.O. Box 1386
Lower Lake, CA 95457
Phone: 707/928-9898
Web site: http://members.aol.com/
yogaresrch

Books

The New Yoga for People Over 50: A Comprehensive Guide for Midlife and Older Beginners, by Suza Francina. 1997. Deerfield Beach, FL. Health Communications, Inc. Paperback. $11.95.
This book contains a section on arthritis.

Relax and Renew: Restful Yoga for Stressful Times, by Judith Lasater. 1995. Berkeley: Rodmell Press. Paperback. $21.95.
A physical therapist and yoga instructor shows how to use pillows and other props for relaxing yoga.

Yoga Journal's Yoga Basics: The Essential Beginner's Guide to Yoga for a Lifetime of Health & Fitness, by Mara Carrico. 1997. New York. Henry Holt and Company, Inc. Paperback. $15.95.

Magazine

Yoga Journal, published bimonthly, also offers an annual list of teachers and many books and videos on yoga. Available on newsstands or can be ordered by calling 800/I-DO-YOGA. Can also be ordered by writing P.O. Box 469088, Escondido, CA 92046-9088 or online at http://www.yogajournal.com.
Single copies: $4.95. One-year subscription (6 issues): $21.95.

Videotapes

There are many yoga videos and they vary widely. Check out the yoga videos at your local library to find one you like, or ask a yoga instructor. Here are some beginner favorites.

Daily Routines for Beginners: Lilias Workout Series. $19.95.

Jane Fonda's Yoga Exercise Workout. $19.95.

Pathways to Better Living with Arthritis with Shoosh Crotzer. $19.50. This video isn't really yoga, but gentle yoga-based exercises. It's recommended by and can be ordered through the Arthritis Foundation by calling 800/207-8633.

Audio Tape

Lilias Complete Yoga. 1994. Audio Renaissance Tapes. $15.95. This three-tape set takes you step by step from beginning yoga to yoga for experienced students. Comes with an illustrated booklet.

Web Sites

Many yoga schools and centers have Web sites.

Yoga Journal
http://www.yogajournal.com

The America Yoga Association
http://members.aol.com/amyogaassn/index.htm.
Contains basic information, and a section called "Using Yoga to Help With Arthritis."

The Yoga Site
http://www.yogasite.com
Has basic information including lists of yoga teachers and places that offer yoga retreats, and a section that summarizes yoga and mind–body research.

Erich Shiffman's
http://www.movingintostillness.com
Has detailed descriptions and photos of basic yoga postures, information on breathing and meditation, and links to many other yoga sites.

There are few studies that look at the effect of yoga on arthritis. A 1994 randomized controlled study in the *Journal of Rheumatology* found yoga practice significantly improved pain, tenderness and finger range of motion for osteoarthritis of the hands (Garfinkel 2). A study that same year in the *British Journal of Rheumatology* suggested yoga is useful for rheumatoid arthritis (Haslock).

Expert Opinion

With the proper practitioner, yoga can be done safely by just about anyone and can be helpful for the symptoms of most kinds of arthritis and related diseases. It yields many of the benefits of meditation and deep relaxation, reducing stress and promoting a glow of well-being that can ease chronic pain and the depression that often accompanies chronic illness.

However, even gentle yoga exercises can be harmful if done incorrectly, so be sure to seek a qualified teacher. Be sure the teacher understands your limitations. Also, yoga does not give the benefits of an aerobic workout.

Finding a Teacher

Although there are no uniform certification standards, individual yoga schools do certify those who complete their teaching programs. Ask a health professional for a referral to a certified teacher. Yoga is taught at many hospitals and health centers, through adult education classes, or at community centers, senior citizen centers and, of course, at yoga centers. *Yoga Journal* (see Resources) publishes a list of teachers every year.

If you have significant pain or movement limitations, look for classes specially designed for your needs. Classes for senior citizens generally feature a more gentle, careful yoga and are a good place to begin.

Cautions

! Be sure to talk with your doctor about any yoga movements or poses you should *not* do. Take a yoga book with pictures of the postures to an appointment, and ask which of the poses or movements you should avoid.

! Tell the yoga instructor about any limitations, painful areas, or concerns you have, and ask if he or she has experience working with these situations.

Good Advice

• Go see a class before you begin. Are you comfortable with the level of the class and the teacher? If the instructor is more interested in perfect poses than in adapting to the limits of each student, this is not the class for you. Also, if the class is taught as a physical workout, without relaxation and breathing exercises, you won't get all the benefits that come with meditative yoga.

Costs

Yoga classes range in cost from around $4 to $20 per session, depending on where you live. There are often discounts for signing up for a block of classes, and for senior citizens. Some health maintenance organizations offer yoga classes at a discount as part of a wellness program.

TAI CHI CHUAN AND QI GONG

Every day, millions of people gather in parks throughout China to practice tai chi chuan or qi gong. To Western eyes, they are performing a series of fitness exercises. But the real purpose of their practice is to balance and enhance their vital life energy, or "qi" (pronounced as chee and often spelled "chi" in the West).

The concept of qi is at the heart of traditional Chinese medicine (see page 33), which believes that disease is due to blocks or imbalances in the flow of qi through the body. Tai chi and qi gong stimulate qi, and are believed to cure illness, strengthen the organs and improve the functioning of all body systems.

Many rheumatologists and physical therapists recommend these gentle movements to patients with muscle and joint diseases. Some tai chi teachers say it is especially good for those with autoimmune diseases such as rheumatoid arthritis, although no controlled studies have shown this to be true.

There are many styles of tai chi and qi gong, and variations within the styles. All are based on meditation and gentle, soft movements taken from the movements of animals or nature. It's considered best to practice at sunrise or sunset outside in nature, so you can absorb the qi of the earth.

Don't try to learn tai chi and qi gong from a video: It's best to learn these practices from a teacher who can explain the philosophy and make sure you are doing the movements correctly. Both are taught in group classes. As you learn the basics, you can practice on your own.

Daily practice is recommended. The practice can take as few as five minutes or can last as long as an hour.

What Happens in a Tai Chi Class

Tai chi can be described as part exercise, part martial art and part spiritual practice. Developed about 600 years ago, it consists of a series of controlled movements that flow rhythmically together into one long, graceful gesture. The sequences have poetic names such as "white stork flaps it wings" or "grasping the bird's tail," and can be beautiful to watch.

Although its roots are in martial arts, tai chi is not violent. The movements are performed slowly and lightly, with concentration and inner stillness. All of your joints should be held softly, never locked or stiffened. Participants wear loose, comfortable clothing and thin-soled shoes or go barefoot.

Tai chi classes usually last about one hour. They begin with warm-up exercises for the body, and then breathing exercises or meditation to quiet the mind. The teacher demonstrates the poses, and the class follows along. The sequences are repeated, focusing

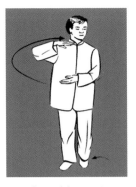

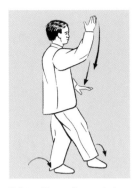

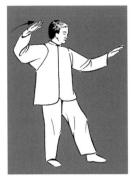

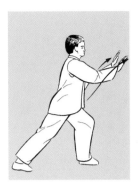

Part the Wild Horse's Mane *(Yema Fenzong)*

White Crane Spreads Its Wings *(Baihe Liangchi)*

Reverse Reeling Forearm *(Daojuan Gong)*

Grasp Sparrow's Tail *(Zuolan Quewel)*

on positions, breathing and inner balance as the class learns them one-by-one.

The long form of tai chi has more than 100 movements and can take 40 minutes to complete. The short version has 24 movements and can take about 10 minutes to complete.

The sequences can be done slowly, or with more speed and energy. But movements are always soft and graceful, a meditation in motion.

What Happens in a Qi Gong Class

Qi gong (spelled many ways such as "chi kung" or "qigong") is much older than tai chi, dating back some 3,000 years. It's a system of meditation, breathing exercises and movements intended to strengthen and direct the flow of qi through the body to promote health and self-healing.

Qi gong has many styles. Some are more active than others, but overall it has fewer movements than tai chi, and is less graceful. Where tai chi poses move fluidly together, qi gong postures are separate movements, each held for a few seconds or longer. Some postures involve only the arms. One of the best known sequences is called "eight brocades," a name meant to describe the movements as strong but as flexible as a piece of brocaded silk.

Those with severe OA of the knees or hips may find qi gong easier to perform than tai chi. The exercises can be done by people of all ages and levels of fitness, even by those in a bed or wheelchair.

A typical qi gong class begins with meditation and breathing techniques to help quiet your mind and body so you can recognize your qi. Teachers say it may take some time before you feel your internal energy. It's been described as a tingling sensation, or as heat or a feeling of fullness. Grand masters of qi gong are said to be able to direct their qi outward to heal others as well.

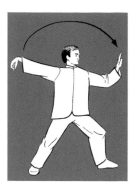

Single Whip (*Danbian*)

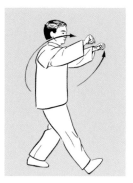

Strike to Ears with Both Fists (*Shuangfeng Guaner*)

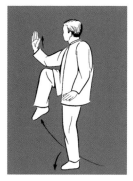

Lower Body and Stand on One Leg (*Zuo Xiashi Duli*)

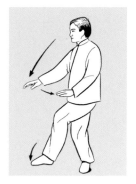

Needle at Sea Bottom (*Haidizhen*)

Scientific Evidence

There are many Chinese studies and reports of the benefits of tai chi and qi gong, but not many English-language ones. The few that there are focus on tai chi. A 1991 study found it appeared safe for patients with rheumatoid arthritis (Kirsteins). Several, including two 1996 studies from the *Journal of the American Geriatric Society* (Wolf, Wolfson) showed tai chi practice significantly decreased the risk of falling for seniors. Study participants also said they felt better.

The effects of qi gong have been studied in Asia, but few English-language studies are available. University of Maryland researchers included qi gong along with mindfulness meditation in a 1998 uncontrolled study for fibromyalgia. Participants said their depression, coping skills, pain threshold and function were significantly improved, both after the study and six months later (Singh).

Expert Opinion

Western doctors may raise an eyebrow at the theories behind qi exercises, but many recommend them for anyone with arthritis and related diseases, especially for seniors. The slow, gentle movements build muscle strength without stressing joints, improve balance, and relieve stress and depression. Qi gong can be done even by those with severely limiting disease because it isn't necessary to move very much to raise one's qi.

Finding a Teacher

It may take some searching to find a qualified teacher in some areas. Check with health, community or senior centers for information about classes. Physical therapists or rehabilitation programs may know of classes, or you can contact a traditional Chinese medicine center. The *Qi Journal* Web site has a list of teachers.

Cautions

! Choose your teacher carefully. There is no uniform certification for teachers. An affiliation with a reputable health center is generally a good sign.

! Never exert yourself doing these exercises. Most teachers believe the internal effects of qi are more important that the physical exercise.

Good Advice

• Because these practices involve your mind as well as your body, only do what feels good to you, both physically and emotionally.

• These disciplines are soft and meditative, and should not be taught as martial arts. Ask the teacher about the goals of the class. If the class focuses on self-defense or hard, violent movements, it is not a tai chi or qi gong class.

Costs

The cost of classes can vary from between $8 and $12, or less if you sign up for a course. Low-cost courses are offered by some health organizations.

ALEXANDER, FELDENKRAIS AND TRAGER

If pain and stiffness are making it hard for you to move, chances are that at least some of your discomfort is being made worse by compensation. You've picked up harmful habits of posture or body use to avoid pain, or to work around a stiff or achy joint.

Pain can "teach" us to hold ourselves and move in ways that stress other parts of the body, setting up an escalating cycle of more pain and function loss. Osteoarthritis pain that's been making you favor your right knee can lead to low back pain. Some scientists think that certain forms of osteoarthritis may even be caused by poor patterns of movement that wear out joints. Chronic pain from fibromyalgia can knot up your muscles and cause tension headaches and temporomandibular joint syndrome.

A course of movement re-education might help. Three of these are the Alexander technique, the Feldenkrais method and the Trager approach, each named for its developer.

All three are based on developing mind–body awareness that helps you recognize old habits of tension and learn new ways of moving. Although each has a unique approach and attitude, all teach how to improve posture, range of motion and breathing; and correct patterns of misuse that can cause pain.

The techniques show you more efficient ways to use damaged joints and sore muscles so that movement and balance take less effort. They relieve joint stress by distributing weight more evenly, and help you feel better by showing you ways to ease pain. All three involve some gentle touching from the instructor to develop body awareness, sometimes as you are lying on a padded table, but these are not forms of massage.

All three of these programs are no sweat – literally. They require minimal exertion, and can be done by anyone at any age or fitness level – from those who are barely mobile to those who are athletically elite.

It's difficult to describe these methods, because they are subtle and the results depend on the interaction between you and the teacher. Although similar in goals, they have different approaches. Some have described them by saying the Alexander technique is a thinking approach, the Feldenkrais method is more physical, and the Trager approach is more intuitive or meditative.

But these are not quick fixes. While most people feel an improvement after even one session, it takes a number of lessons over time to change life-long habits and to retrain your mind, muscles and nervous system to move your body more easily. With practice, you can expect to feel more comfortable in your body, to be more stable and to move more freely.

After a few weeks of these classes, you may be ready to do yoga, tai chi, dance and other exercise with much less pain.

What Happens in an Alexander Session

This technique emphasizes balancing and aligning the head, neck and spine to allow the body to move more efficiently. It was devised by F. Mathias Alexander (1869–1955), an actor with chronic laryngitis. By observing and working on himself, he discovered his throat problem was caused by tension and poor movement habits. He developed a system of lessons to help correct this and other neuromuscular malfunctions.

Alexander technique is taught one-on-one in private lessons of 30–45 minutes, where the teacher can work with an individual situation and give immediate feedback. Using a guiding touch and instructions, Alexander teachers bring your awareness to poor posture and habits of misuse that lead to inefficient and even harmful patterns of holding and moving the body. Part of the lesson takes place on a padded table, and part involves showing you how to improve everyday functions: Students learn to walk, stand, and sit without strain, and to improve work habits.

Alexander technique can have an immediate practical use: You might notice for the first time how the way you carry your head and neck stresses your back, or how tension around your inflamed hip affects your balance. People who hate exercise often like Alexander because there are no "exercises": The technique is intended to be used in everyday awareness and activities.

The number of lessons depends on your situation and personal goals, but a recommended course is 30 private sessions, usually taken twice a week. Some students return every year or so for a "tune-up."

What Happens in a Feldenkrais Session

The Feldenkrais method uses a program of subtle movements to help you become aware of your body, discover how your body moves, and to explore new movement skills. Moshe Feldenkrais (1904–1984) a physicist, engineer and martial arts expert, developed his method to overcome an old knee injury.

The method is taught both one-on-one and in classes. In the hour-long classes, called "Awareness Through Movement," a practitioner guides a group through a sequence of very small, non-stressful movements meant to increase body awareness, flexibility and range of motion. These sessions usually begin with students lying on floor mats, moving one set of muscles at a time, but exercises are also done standing and sitting as students discover more comfortable ways to move.

During the individual lessons, called "Functional Integration," the student sits or lies on a table and the practitioner gently moves his or her body through a series of movements, discovering the range of motion and allowing the student to experience free movement on a conscious and unconscious level. Sessions usually last about an hour.

A private session followed by a six-week series of classes twice a week is recommended, with an occasional "tune-up" workshop after that. Students can do exercises on their own at home after learning the basics, but many like to attend classes as well.

What Happens in a Trager Session

Trager practitioners believe pain and stress begin in the mind, and that working on the body allows us to access and change both physical and mental patterns. The method was developed by Milton Trager, MD (1908–1997), a boxer and fitness buff who earned a medical degree in middle-age.

Trager therapists work in a deeply meditative state, using touch and gentle exercises to communicate with the client's unconscious. In Trager table work, you lie, loosely clothed or in underwear, on a padded table. The practitioner gently moves your body, rhythmically rocking, stretching, or taking the joints and muscles through range of motion, helping you experience what it feels like to relax and let go of tension and stress. The gentle manipulative movements enter both the conscious and unconscious mind, changing the mental and

physical experience of movement to that of relaxation and pleasure rather than pain. Private sessions last about an hour and a half each. The number of sessions depends on your situation and response: You may require four sessions, or weekly sessions for several months.

A system of gentle, freeform movement sequences called "Mentastics" (which stands for mental gymnastics) helps increase body–mind awareness and range of motion. There are many Mentastic sequences, some as small as shifting weight from one side to another, others that involve full-body, dance-like movements. Mentastics can be included in your sessions with table work, or given in classes. There is no set number of classes recommended, and the exercises can be practiced alone, once the concept is learned.

Scientific Evidence

There are few studies of these techniques that pass scientific scrutiny and none we could find for arthritis. However, physical therapists have written about the benefits of all three for osteoarthritis, rheumatoid arthritis and fibromyalgia.

The Alexander technique is best documented. A 1999 controlled study in the *Journal of Gerontology: Medical Sciences* showed it improved both balance and functional reach in a group of older women (Dennis). In a controlled 1988 study of breathing function in healthy adults, 20 Alexander lessons improved chest muscle function (Austin). In an uncontrolled study that year, participants in a multidisciplinary pain management program said the Alexander technique helped more with chronic pain than several other relaxation or exercise programs they had tried (Fisher).

An uncontrolled study that looked at the Trager approach and 12 people with chronic lung disease found some lung function measurements improved after two weeks of treatments (Witt).

Expert Opinion

These programs may be useful, and have little risk. They offer a different approach to moving, and the concentrated one-on-one sessions sometimes show you more than many exercise sessions. In fact, physical therapists and doctors refer patients to these programs, and they are included in some rehabilitation programs. The movements are gentle and generally safe for everyone.

But not everyone will have the patience to persist and the time it takes to do these programs, or be willing to pay for them.

Finding a Therapist

Legitimate therapists in these disciplines are all trained and certified by the organizations. There about 1,000 certified Alexander technique teachers in the United States; about 1,500 practitioners certified by The Feldenkrais Guild; and about 750 practitioners listed through and certified by the Trager Institute.

Cautions

! Although these therapies are generally safe, pay attention to your body and don't do anything that hurts.

Good Advice

• Although even a few sessions will show you some better ways to use your body, you need to commit to a program of classes and practice to reap the most benefit.

Costs

These movement re-education therapies are not generally covered by insurance, but may be if given by a physical therapist or prescribed by a physician. Some health plans may cover these programs or offer them at reduced rates. Private session rates vary from $40 to $90. Group classes are about $10 per class.

Organizations

North American Society of Teachers of the Alexander Technique
401 East Market Street
Charlottesville, VA 22902
Phone: 800/473-0620
E-mail: nastat@ix.netcom.com
Web site: http://www.alexandertech.org

Alexander Technique International
1692 Massachusetts Avenue, Third Floor
Cambridge, MA 02138
Phone: 888/321-0856
E-mail: usa@ati-net.com
Web site: http://www.ati-net.com

The Feldenkrais Guild of North America (FGNA)
524 Ellsworth Street SW
Albany, OR 97321-0143
Phone: 800/775-2118
E-mail: feldngld@peak.org
Web site: http//www.feldenkrais.com

The Trager Institute
21 Locust Avenue
Mill Valley, CA 94941-2806
Phone: 415/388-2688
E-mail: admin@trager.com
Web site: http://www.trager.com

Books

Awareness Heals: The Feldenkrais Method for Dynamic Health, by Steven Shafarman. 1997. Reading, MA. Addison Wesley Longman Publishing Company, Inc. Paperback. $14.

Body Learning: An Introduction to the Alexander Technique, by Michael J. Gelb. 1996. New York. Henry Holt & Company. Paperback. $10.95.

Moving Medicine: The LifeWork of Milton Trager, MD, by Jack Liskin. 1995. Station Hill Press. Hardcover. $24.95.

Videotape

First Lesson: An Introduction to the Alexander Technique with William Hurt and Jane Kosminsky. $49.96. Order from Balance of Well-Being: 888/881-1902.

Web Site

"Alleviating Arthritis Pain and Discomfort: How the Alexander Technique Can Help," by Glenna Batson, physical therapist and associate professor of anatomy-kinesiology at the University of North Carolina, Chapel Hill, can be found on her Web site at http://www.glennabatson.com

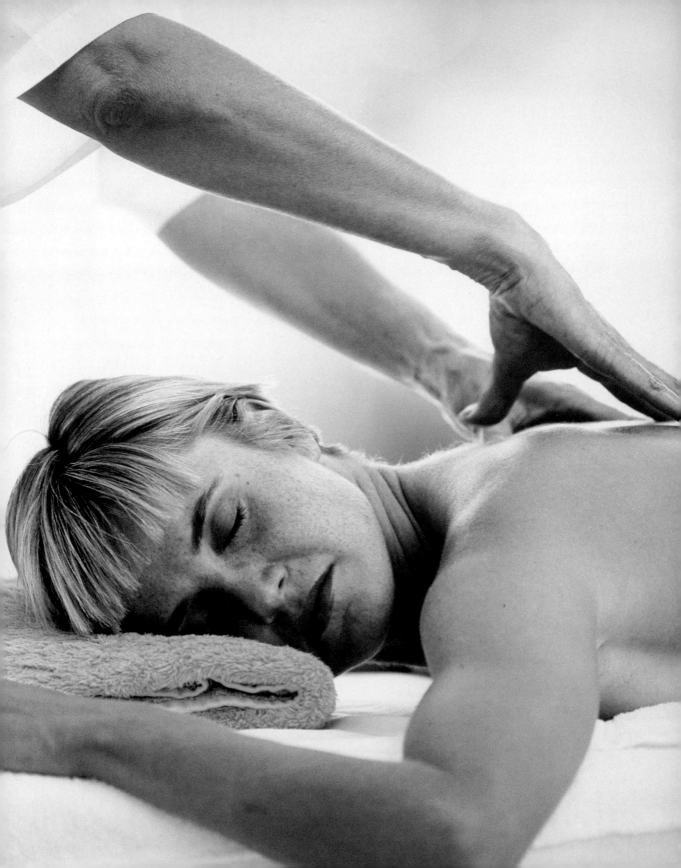

Massage and Bodywork

The Healing Power of Touch

A word on definitions: *Massage* is usually defined as a manipulation of the soft tissue, using pressure, stroking and so on. Many hands-on therapies use other techniques, so we've used the term *bodywork* as a broader term to describe all types of touch therapy.

The healing power of touch has been used since antiquity to maintain health and ease the pains of body, mind and soul. It comes naturally to most of us, in the soothing strokes and pats we receive as babies and later give to others as signs of sympathy and comfort.

In just about every culture, there is a tradition of using the hands as therapeutic tools, and for those with chronic musculoskeletal diseases such as arthritis, manual therapy can have many physical and emotional benefits. It can help stretch tight muscles, improve flexibility, and break the cycle of pain, stress and depression that accompanies chronic illness. What's more, it feels good. But the Puritan roots run deep in some of us: Although we willingly endure many uncomfortable and even unpleasant therapies for the sake of our health, many of us have a hard time investing in something that seems more like a luxury than a medical treatment.

That's not true in many other cultures, where massage is part of the established medical system. It is one of the basic treatments of Indian ayurvedic medicine (see page 29). In China, whole medical departments in major hospitals are devoted to massage. It is an accepted medical therapy in many European countries, especially in Middle and Eastern Europe, as well as the former Soviet Union.

Massage used to be part of the U.S. medical system as well. It was used by doctors into the early 20th century. Then the development of modern medical technology made it seem old-fashioned and too time-consuming. It didn't give the dramatic and consistent results of drugs or surgery, and it gradually faded out of conventional medical practice.

Today, massage and other manual therapies are making a comeback in medicine. Massage is among the most-used complementary therapies (Eisenberg). Many rehabilitation programs and chronic pain clinics include a bodywork therapist as part of the treatment team, and rheumatologists often recommend massage for arthritis and related diseases. A 1998 national survey of 1,007 people conducted by the American Massage Therapy Association showed 22 percent of those interviewed had a massage within the past five years, and 13 percent within the past year. Massage may also have your doctor's approval. Of those who discussed massage with their doctors, 76 percent reported a favorable response.

A QUICK GUIDE TO BODYWORK

There are more than 100 types of body-work, each with its own technique and philosophy. They offer similar physical, emotional – and in some cases spiritual – benefits for those with arthritis and related diseases. But they have different approaches.

Some types, such as Swedish massage, emphasize the physical, using pressing, rubbing and manipulation to work on muscles and joints to improve function. Asian techniques emphasize balancing the flow of vital energy in your body. And some – such as reiki and therapeutic touch – focus on energy for spiritual healing, and practitioners don't physically touch you at all.

The list below gives a description of some of the more common bodywork types and how they might help with arthritis. Thomas Claire's book *Bodywork* gives detailed descriptions of many types and techniques (see Resources). Some types will appeal to you more than others, and these descriptions can help you decide what kind of approach you might want. If you decide to try massage, don't get too hung up on the names and types of techniques. Competent massage therapists are trained in many techniques. It's best to tell a practitioner what effect you'd like to get from the treatment, or what symptoms you want to relieve, and let the expert choose the best therapy.

Western Massage

These massage styles are among the best known, most often practiced and most researched in the United States. These techniques are used to relieve pain, stress, tension, depression and fatigue. Often a practitioner will include several of these techniques in an "eclectic" style to suit your individual needs.

You don't have to completely disrobe for a massage, but it's common to take off most clothing, for comfort, to allow the therapist to have direct contact with your skin, and to prevent stains from oils or lotions. However, you only need to remove as much clothing as feels comfortable. You certainly don't need to undress beyond your underwear, and you can tell the therapist to limit the massage to specific areas such as your back, legs and so on.

Swedish Massage

Swedish massage or European massage is what most of us think of as massage. It's a full-body treatment that involves stroking or kneading the top layers of muscles with oils or lotions. It's usually given as a one-hour treatment, and can have varied effects. It can be a soothing way to relieve muscle tension and promote relaxation, or it can be quite vigorous. It's a good introduction to

For Those Who Don't Want a Full-Body Massage

The idea of being kneaded like bread dough may not appeal to you. Or you may hurt so much you can't imagine anyone rubbing your aching body. Or you may not want to take off your clothes. You can still get the relaxation and pain-relief benefits of massage if you limit touch to specific body areas. Two therapies you might consider are reflexology and CranioSacral Therapy.™

Reflexology therapy massages points on the feet, hands or ears that are believed to correspond to organs or other body parts. The technique probably originated with acupressure (see page 135). But the theory behind foot and hand reflexology – the technique most practiced in the United States – is a modern one based on a concept of vertical energy channels that run from your extremities up through the body. Your feet and hands are rich in nerve endings, so it's possible that stimulating them could have effects on other parts of your body. Whatever the theory, many find gentle massage of the feet or hands relaxing.

A randomized, placebo-controlled study looked at 38 women with premenstrual syndrome (PMS) who got either true reflexology or a sham reflexology treatment. Those who received true reflexology had a significantly greater decreases in symptoms (Oleson).

There have been no studies directly relating to arthritis. Although there are not studies to prove this, it may help improve circulation for those with Raynaud's phenomenon and ease stiffness from osteoarthritis and rheumatoid arthritis.

CranioSacral Therapy™ uses a gentle manipulation meant to balance the fluids in the craniosacral system that runs from your skull (cranio) down to the base of your spine (sacrum). The practitioner stands behind you while you lie on a table, gently cradling your skull in his or her hands and applying very light pressure to purportedly affect the flow of fluids in the system or to "adjust" the bones of the skull. There may be some pressure placed on the sacrum, the bones at the base of your spine, as well.

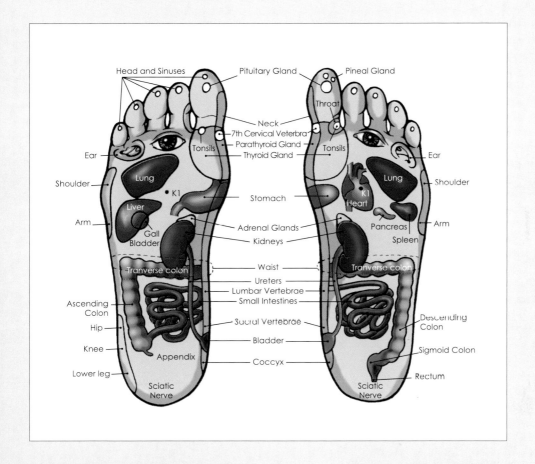

Head and Sinuses · Pituitary Gland · Pineal Gland · Throat · Neck · 7th Cervical Veterbra · Parathyroid Gland · Tonsils · Thyroid Gland · Ear · Shoulder · Lung · K1 · Liver · Arm · Gall Bladder · Stomach · Adrenal Glands · Kidneys · Heart · Pancreas · Spleen · Tranverse colon · Waist · Ureters · Lumbar Vertebrae · Small Intestines · Ascending Colon · Hip · Sacral Vertebrae · Descending Colon · Knee · Bladder · Appendix · Coccyx · Sigmoid Colon · Lower leg · Rectum · Sciatic Nerve

There's controversy over whether this technique has any validity at all (Rogers 1, Rogers 2). Experts debate whether there is a craniosacral system and whether the bones of the skull, which fuse together in adults, can be manipulated. However, there are many anecdotes of those who say it helps. Help or not, it is safe. For those with arthritis or related conditions, this may ease pain, particularly headache, and help you experience relaxation.

massage, especially for those with a lot of pain from RA, fibromyalgia or other conditions because it can be quite gentle and help promote relaxation.

Deep Tissue Massage

Deep tissue massage, as the name says, uses strong pressure on deep muscle or tissue layers to relieve chronic tension. Often the strokes go across the grain of the muscles and the therapist will use fingers, thumbs and even elbows. This can cause some soreness, especially in the first sessions, and is not for everyone. It can help with the tight muscles associated with guarding and favoring arthritic joints. It also is often used to relieve low back pain.

Trigger Point Therapy

Trigger point therapy (sometimes called neuromuscular massage) uses deep finger pressure on specific spots to release trigger points: knots of tension or pain that can "trigger" pain in other parts of the body. It's said that President John Kennedy attributed his rehabilitation from debilitating back pain to this therapy, which was developed by his physician, Janet Travell, MD. It may be particularly helpful for fibromyalgia, but it can also be very painful if the pressure is too strong. You and your therapist have to be aware of you body's response to this technique. You might want to start off with a more soothing, overall massage to relax the muscles first.

Myofascial Release

Myofascial release works on relieving tension in the fascia, the thin connective tissue that sheaths your muscles. Therapists use slow, fairly gentle but steady pressure to stretch the fascia. Sessions last about 30 minutes, and no oil is used. It's used for fibromyalgia, chronic pain and stress, and is said to release emotional tightness as well.

Oriental Bodywork and Massage

Bodywork techniques from Asia are close relatives of acupuncture (see page 135). They are based on the theory that blockages or imbalances in the flow of vital life energy, or qi (pronounced chee), produce illness. Pressure or massage on acupuncture points can balance the flow of qi and improve health.

You can wear loose clothing for these treatments. They are recommended for improving energy levels, relieving stress and pain, and improving sleep.

Acupressure Massage

Acupressure massage works like acupuncture, using finger and hand pressure instead of needles to unblock or balance your qi. Many Western massage styles use acupressure techniques along with massage (see What Happens in an Acupressure Treatment, page 138). Shiatsu is a Japanese version of acupressure. It also works on balancing energy flow, called ki (pronounced kee) in Japan. Specific points similar

Skinrolling Massage and Spray and Stretch

Two specialized techniques for fibromyalgia

Skinrolling massage is a technique that has had good results for some with fibromyalgia – but isn't very widely known. Be warned: It can be very painful at first, so painful some need a mild anesthetic for the first sessions. Basically, the practitioner picks up a roll of your skin and moves it across the underlying fascia to break adhesions that painfully bind tissue layers and nerve connections that are communicating pain. Those with skin-fold tenderness who have been able to stand the pain of the first few procedures say they have had dramatic and long-lasting pain relief. But if it's too painful, you can ask the therapist to stop at any time (Hirschberg).

The technique is used in Europe, but you may have difficulty finding a practitioner in the United States.

Spray and Stretch is another unconventional technique. Physical therapists are divided about this technique and there are no studies that show its effectiveness. But here again, many say it has helped.

A coolant, such as flouri-methane, is sprayed over a painful area to anesthetize it. Then the muscles in that area are stretched gently by the therapist. This technique is most often performed by a physician or a physical therapist. If you decide to try it, make sure the therapist has experience with the technique. If you don't feel better a day or so after trying either of these therapies, they may not be right for you.

to acupuncture points are pressed and held. Sessions are given on a mat on the floor, and can include stretching and massage as well as acupressure. Tuina (tway-nah), a traditional Chinese medicine massage that includes pres-sure point massage, is just gaining popularity in the United States.

There aren't many acupressure studies reported in English, or many good controlled studies. Acupuncture, which stimulates the

Getting the Most Out of Bodywork

- Decide what you want. Before you book a bodywork session, think about your goals: Do you want to try a specific technique or school of bodywork? Do you want a soothing massage to relieve stress, or do you want more vigorous work on a specific part of your body? Will you be more comfortable with a male or female therapist?

- Choose an experienced practitioner. People with chronic ailments need practitioners who know how to work with that condition. Ask the therapist about his or her experience, and look for one who has experience working with your particular health condition.

- Prepare for the session. Bathe or shower earlier the same day you plan a bodywork session, and don't eat or drink alcohol for a few hours before and afterward. Schedule enough time so you don't have to hurry away when you're done.

- Talk to the therapist. If you are new to this kind of bodywork, ask what to expect. State your preferences about music, lights, incense, and if you want to talk or be silent during the session. Say how strongly or gently you want to be touched. Tell the therapist about sensitive areas, or places you don't want to be touched, and speak up immediately if anything is painful or uncomfortable at any time.

- Keep the glow. Remain resting for a few minutes after the session. If possible, avoid plunging back into a hectic situation. That way, you can enjoy the peaceful feeling longer. Drink lots of fluids: Therapists say bodywork promotes circulation, and water will help flush out the toxins. Avoid caffeine or alcohol for a few hours, because these substances alter your physical and mental responses.

same points, has been shown to relieve pain from osteoarthritis (Christensen) and fibromyalgia (DeLuze, Sprott). But the same results may not apply to acupressure.

Structural Integration Bodywork

These techniques work at improving your function by treating underlying problems with muscles or bone alignment. They can help you move more easily and can relieve pain caused by imbalances in your body structure. Often, practitioners will use massage techniques along with these.

Chiropractic adjustment and osteopathic manipulation are among the best known of these therapies. They are discussed in the chapter Alternative Healing Systems (page 27).

Rolfing

Rolfing is named for Ida P. Rolf, who developed techniques to "restructure" the body. It uses techniques similar to deep tissue massage to release fascia tightness caused by injury, stress or habits of misuse. The aim of Rolfing is to release muscles and other tissues from the fascia, a flexible sheath of connective tissue that covers the muscles, and allow the body to better align itself. No oil is used, so the therapist can better connect with the muscles. The therapy is given in 10 one-hour sessions about a week apart. Treatments are aimed at improving function rather than treating disease, with the idea that improved function will put less wear and tear on your joints.

There aren't any studies that prove this, however. One randomized, controlled study that tested anxiety scores before and five weeks after Rolfing found reduced anxiety in those who had received the therapy (Weinberg). An uncontrolled study of 10 patients with cerebral palsy who underwent Rolfing had mixed results. Those with mild impairment were able to walk faster, those with moderate impairment improved only slightly, and those with severe disease showed no improvement. Moreover, all had increased muscle tightness that the researcher thought could outweigh any other benefits (Perry).

A similar approach is Hellerwork, an offshoot of Rolfing that includes exercises and movement re-education. Other methods that focus on correcting movement, (but use very gentle touching) are the Alexander technique, Feldenkrais method and the Trager approach (see Moving Medicine, page 97).

Western Energy Therapies

There are several Western bodywork techniques that are based on enhancing and balancing vital life energy. However, these practices don't use acupuncture points. They are related more to ancient "laying on of the hands." No one knows how they work, and there are few studies and little scientific evidence. Because there is little or no actual touching, these treatments are safe and may appeal to those in extreme pain who can't stand to be touched.

Polarity Therapy

Polarity therapy is based on the theory that the body contains both positive and negative currents of energy that need to be in balance for good health. The practitioner uses a gentle touch to hold key points in your "energy anatomy" to help remove blocks and to balance energy. He or she may also use some gentle massage techniques. It's intended to promote health, not diagnose or treat diseases. Sessions last from 60 to 90 minutes, and treatment can include advice on diet and lifestyle. We found no studies that showed the effect of polarity therapy on arthritis.

Therapeutic Touch

Therapeutic touch isn't really touch at all, because practitioners don't make contact with the body. It's based on the theory that we have energy fields that extend beyond our physical bodies. Entering a meditative state, a practitioner uses his or her hands to feel problems in another person's energy field, and channel universal energy to help heal disease and ease pain. This very unconventional therapy was developed within the U.S. medical system in the 1970s, and popularized by a nurse named Delores Krieger. It's very popular among nurses, and is taught in more than 80 universities. Sessions last about 30 minutes, and fees are based on the ability to pay.

Therapeutic touch has gotten mixed reviews. A 1998 single-blind, randomized, controlled study of 25 patients with osteoarthritis of the knee compared therapeutic touch, mock therapeutic touch and standard care. Those who got the real therapeutic touch had significantly decreased pain and improved function compared to the other two groups (Gordon). However, a study earlier that year questioned the whole basis of therapeutic touch: It found practitioners were only able to detect a human energy field 44 percent of the time, less than by chance alone (Rosa).

Reiki

Reiki (pronounced ray-key) means "spiritually guided universal life energy" in Japanese. The practitioner channels this spiritual energy into the person being treated. It involves little or no actual contact with the patient's body. The energy balances or enhances the recipient's own life energy to promote healing. Advocates claim it can relieve symptoms of chronic disease, including arthritis and lupus. Sessions last 60–90 minutes. A 1997 uncontrolled pilot study of 20 patients with various kinds of pain showed a significant reduction in pain (Olson).

What Happens in a Bodywork Session

Sessions vary depending on whether you are having a massage or some other treatment. However, your session will most likely be given on a padded table or a mat on the floor in a warm, quiet room. It may be softy lit, with quiet music and incense (the therapist will ask your preferences about light and music); or it may be more like a typical doctor's office. Before beginning treatment, the

Do-It-Yourself Massage

It's natural. When something hurts, we rub or squeeze it. And, usually, the sore spot feels a bit better. With a little practice and some advice from a massage therapist, you can turn that instinct into do-it-yourself massage. It's not as relaxing as having someone else work on you, but it can help ease pain and tension. And it will give you double benefits: The part you are massaging will feel better, and so will your hands that are doing the work.

Conditions that may particularly benefit – and are easy to reach – include osteoarthritis aches in knees and ankles, and hands with rheumatoid arthritis and Raynaud's phenomenon.

Some tips for a good self-massage:

- Ask a professional for advice. A massage therapist who has worked on your body can show you some techniques to use yourself.

- Warm up before you begin. A warm bath or shower relaxes you and improves circulation.

- Create a healing setting. Find a warm, quiet place where you won't be disturbed. Music may also set the mood for relaxation.

- Use a little oil or lotion. A lightly-scented massage oil will soothe your spirit as well as your body. Sesame oil is used for massages in Ayurveda, the traditional medical system of India (see page 29). Or you might want to use a lotion made with capsicum (see page 197) or another pain-reliever. (Do be sure to wash carefully after you use capsicum, to avoid spreading it to your eyes or other sensitive tissues.)

- Consider a massage appliance. Vibrating massages can be especially useful if your hand movement is limited or painful, or for hard-to-reach places. Follow instructions, and limit the appliance use to a few minutes at a time. Don't go overboard.

- Use firm but gentle strokes and pressure, especially over your joints where the skin and muscle layers are thin. Pressing or rubbing too hard can irritate your skin and the joint or muscle you are trying to relax.

Organizations

The National Certification Board for Therapeutic Massage and Bodywork
8201 Greensboro Drive, Suite 300
McLean, VA 22102
Phone: 800/296-0664 or 703/610-9015
E-mail: mswiscoski@ncbtmb.org
Web site: http://www.ncbtmc.com
The NCBTMB has a referral list.

The American Massage Therapy Association
820 Davis Street, Suite 100
Evanston, IL 60201
Phone: 847/864-0123
E-mail: info@inet.amtamassage.org
Web site: http://www.amtamassage.org/massagetherapy.htm
The site has good information and articles about massage. Its locator service can direct you to a therapist in your area.

Touch Research Institute
Department of Pediatrics
University of Miami School of Medicine
P.O. Box 016820 (Dept. 820)
1601 NW 12th Avenue
Miami, FL 33101
Phone: 305/243-6781
E-mail: tfield@mednet.med.miami.edu or field@nsu.nova.edu
Web site: http://www.Miami.edu/touch-research
This research group has many articles and studies on its Web site.

MFR(Myofascial Release) Center & Seminars
222 West Lancaster Avenue
Paoli, PA 19301
Phone: 610/644-0136
Web site: http://www.vll.com\mfr

American Polarity Therapy Association
288 Bluff Street, Suite 149
Boulder, CO 80301
Phone: 303/545-2080
E-mail: hq@polaritytherapy.org
Web site: http://www.polaritytherapy.org
Certifies practitioners and has a directory of members.

The International Center for Reiki Training
21421 Hilltop Street, Unit #28
Southfield, MI 48034
Phone: 800/332-8112
Web site: http://www.reiki.org

The Rolf Institute of Structural Integration
205 Canyon Boulevard
Boulder, CO 80302
Phone: 800/530-8875 or 303/449-5903
E-mail: RolfInst@rolf.org
Web site: http://www.rolf.org

Books

Better Health with Foot Reflexology, by Dwight C. Byers. 1991. St. Petersburg, FL. Ingham Publishing, Inc. Hardcover. $24.95.

Bodywork: What Type of Massage to Get - And How to Make the Most of It, by Thomas Claire. 1995. New York. William Morrow & Company. Paperback. $15.

CranioSacral Therapy, Somatoemotional Release, Your Inner Physician and You, by John E. Upledger, DO. 1997. North Atlantic Books. Paperback. $14.95.

Discovering the Body's Wisdom, by Mirka Knaster. 1996. Bantam Books. Paperback. $15.95.

Empowerment Through Reiki: Path to Personal and Global Transformation, by Paula Horan. 1998. Lotus Light Publications. Paperback. $14.95.

Healing Massage Techniques: Holistic, Classic, and Emerging Methods, by Frances M. Tappan. 1988. Appleton & Lange. Paperback. $29.95.

Rolfing: Reestablishing the Natural Alignment and Structural Integration of the Human Body for Vitality and Well-Being, by Ida P. Rolf. 1990. Inner Traditions Int. Ltd. Paperback. $24.95.

The Therapeutic Touch: How to Use Your Hands to Heal, by Dolores Krieger. 1991. New York. Simon & Schuster. Paperback. $11.

Travell and Simons' Myofascial Pain and Dysfunction: The Trigger Point Manual, by Janet G. Travell, MD, David G. Simons, MD, and Lois S. Simons. 1998. Baltimore. Lippincott Williams and Wilkins. Hardcover. $189.
This is a textbook intended for the professional.

Videotape

Massage for Health shows how to perform a simple therapeutic massage. It features Shari Belafonte-Harper and is demonstrated by professional massage therapists Mirka Knaster and James Heartland. Healing Arts Video. $14.99.

therapist will talk to you about any special health conditions or sensitivities, and discuss your goals for the session.

You don't have to disrobe completely: For Oriental bodywork and Western energy therapies, you can wear loose, comfortable clothing. However, for most full-body massages, it's best to remove all or most of your clothing for comfort and to prevent stains from oils or lotions. You'll be given privacy to disrobe and a large sheet to cover yourself. As the therapist massages you, only the part of your body that is being worked on is uncovered.

Most sessions last about an hour or an hour and a half. The practitioner will encourage you to let go of tension, and to concentrate on the bodywork experience and your physical, mental and emotional responses. During the session, the therapist will remind you to breathe, and will move you or tell you what to do. Speak up at anytime if you are ill-at-ease, uncomfortable, or have any questions. Many people relax completely. Some even fall asleep during a massage. You may have an emotional release as well: You may feel tears well up as your body and mind relax.

Bodywork should not hurt, unless you are having a specialized treatment such as deep tissue work. Afterward, you should feel relaxed but energized. You may have some soreness if a stiff joint or tender area has been worked, but that should disappear over the next day. To see some benefits, practitioners generally suggest you try four to six sessions about a week apart.

Scientific Evidence

Massage advocates tend to say that bodywork is good for just about anything that ails you. That may be an overstatement, but studies show it decreases stress hormones and depression, eases muscle pain and spasms, increases pain-killing endorphins and improves sleep and immune function.

A key benefit of massage for many is that it renews the mind–body connection by promoting relaxation. When the main message you've been getting from your body is pain, massage can remind you what it feels like to relax and let go of pain. It may also help you learn how to control pain through relaxation.

The Touch Research Institute (TRI) at the University of Miami School of Medicine has been studying the effects of massage and other touch therapies since 1982. One of its studies showing the basic value of massage found that premature babies who were gently massaged daily gained nearly 50 percent more weight, were more active and were able to leave the hospital sooner than babies who didn't get touched (Field 1).

A TRI randomized, placebo-controlled study of the effects of massage on fibromyalgia compared Swedish massage, TENS (transcutaneous electrical nerve stimulation) and a sham TENS treatment over a five-week period (Sun-

shine). People in the massage group showed improvement in their fibromyalgia symptoms including insomnia, pain, fatigue, anxiety and depression. They also showed lowered cortisol (a hormone involved in the stress response) levels immediately after the sessions. The true TENS group showed similar changes, but only after the last day of the study; the sham TENS group showed no changes.

Another randomized, controlled trial compared massage and TENS for 20 women with chronic fatigue syndrome (Field 2). The women who got massages twice weekly for five weeks had significantly better improvement than the TENS group in many of the symptoms of chronic fatigue syndrome, including pain, depression and sleeplessness. They also tested for decreased urine and saliva cortisol levels.

A 1997 controlled study of children with juvenile rheumatoid arthritis compared massage with relaxation therapy. Children who were massaged for 15 minutes a day by their parents for 30 days had lower stress hormone levels and less pain and morning stiffness than the group participating in relaxation therapy (Field 3).

One study suggests massage improves immune system functioning. A 1996 study of HIV-positive men who had daily massages for a month showed a significant increase in their natural killer cells, the immune system's first line of defense (Ironson). However, there were no changes in other markers of HIV disease progression, such as CD4 counts.

Expert Opinion

There's plenty of evidence to show that when performed by an experienced practitioner, Swedish and Western massage can ease pain and stress.

If you feel better after a treatment, massage may be a useful addition to your regular therapy. People who are isolated or depressed may get an extra benefit from the caring human interaction and the non-sexual, non-threatening intimacy. Relieving aches and stiffness may also make it easier for you to start an exercise routine, which has many of the benefits of massage and in addition builds muscle strength and endurance.

However, massage can be expensive, it is not usually covered by insurance, and the effects may not be lasting. Massage is not harmless: You are putting yourself into some very powerful hands, so be sure to consult a qualified practitioner.

Finding a Therapist

You can find bodywork therapists through professional organizations (see page 128) or through health clinics, rehabilitation programs and pain centers. Ask your physician or other health professionals for a referral, or ask your friends: Word of mouth is a good way to find a therapist. Physical therapists and chiro-

practors often work with massage therapists or can refer you to one. Health clubs and spas also feature massage and bodywork. In general, the Yellow Pages and classifieds are not good places to look unless the therapist is clearly affiliated with a legitimate professional or medical organization.

Massage therapists are required to be licensed in at least 28 states and the District of Columbia. The National Certification Board for Therapeutic Massage and Bodywork (NCBTMB) has certified more than 35,000 massage therapists and has a referral service (see Resources).

Practitioners of other bodywork types are not generally required to be licensed, but most good therapists are certified by a school or through a professional organization. Standards may vary, so be sure to ask about training and certification.

Cautions

! Bodywork is generally safe, but there are some types that might not be appropriate for you. Talk to your doctor first if you have rheumatoid arthritis, ankylosing spondylitis or osteoporosis. He or she may be able to refer you to a practitioner or give you specific cautions.

! Don't have bodywork or massage on inflamed joints, or if you are having a flare, have a fever, have an infection, or are coming down with an acute illness. It may make these worse.

! Don't have massage on areas where your skin is broken, sore or where it hurts. Massage should not be painful.

! Consult your doctor if you have metastatic cancer, high blood pressure or osteoporosis; or if you have varicose veins, phlebitis or other circulation problems. Some massage techniques could make these worse.

! If you are pregnant be sure to tell the practitioner. Certain techniques may contribute to a miscarriage.

! Be aware that these techniques tap into the mind and emotions, and may bring up powerful feelings. Most often, these are feelings of peace and relaxation. But you may also experience sadness or even tears. If strong emotions continue to surface, you may want to seek counseling.

Good Advice

• The type of bodywork you choose doesn't matter as much as your interaction with the therapist. Choose a skilled therapist with experience treating your kind of condition. You need to be able to trust the therapist and relax to get the most benefit from the therapy. You may not feel comfortable being touched by some people – trust your instincts. Many therapists are trained in a number of bodywork or massage techniques, so they can create a treatment for your specific needs.

• Ask if your health provider or insurer covers massage *before* you go for a treatment. It may be offered at a reduced rate through your provider, or covered if prescribed by your physician.

• Bodywork can make you feel vulnerable. Communicate with the therapist, stating your preferences or your dislikes.

• The therapist's touch should always be non-sexual and non-threatening, and you should feel safe and comfortable with the therapist. If at any time you feel ill-at-ease, physically uncomfortable or in pain, tell the therapist. If your feelings continue, don't be shy about stopping in the middle of a session and leaving.

Costs

Bodywork prices vary widely by type and by region. The range is from $30 to $125 or more for an hour. Some practitioners give discounts to clients who book regular appointments. Treatment is often covered by health insurance, especially if prescribed by a doctor or given by a physical therapist, but the number of sessions covered may be limited.

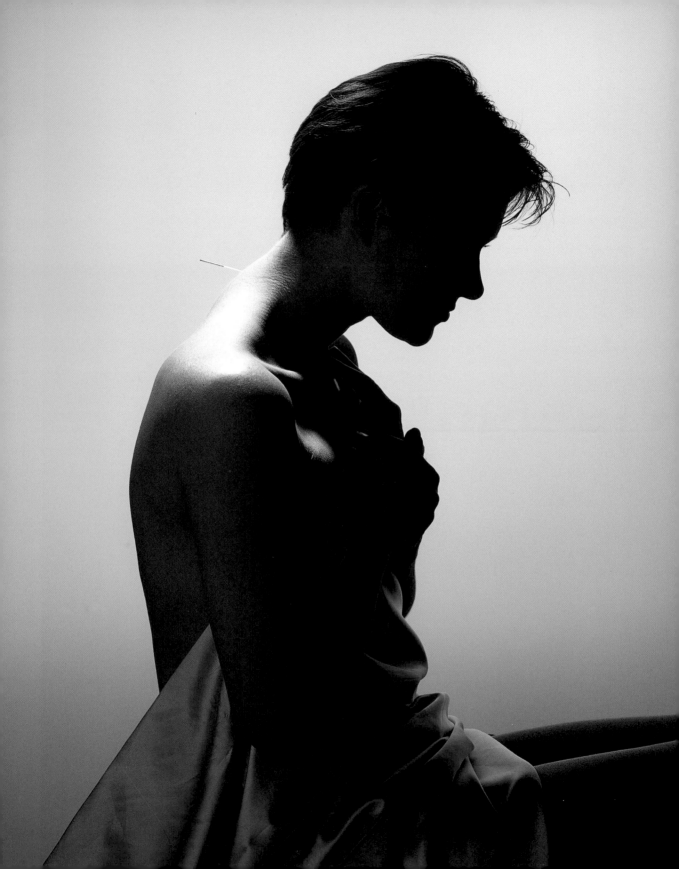

Acupuncture And Acupressure

STIMULATING ENERGY POINTS

Acupuncture is used by hundreds of millions of people around the world to treat almost every ailment. Now it's easing into the mainstream of Western medicine as an increasing number of Americans try this ancient Chinese practice.

More than 15 million Americans have used acupuncture, primarily for pain relief. And because pain is the number one symptom that troubles people with arthritis, acupuncture is being used to treat many kinds of arthritis including osteoarthritis, rheumatoid arthritis, fibromyalgia, gout and Raynaud's phenomenon. Proponents say acupuncture can give significant pain relief, especially when other treatments haven't worked. It has become a key treatment in many chronic pain programs and clinics.

For more than 2,500 years, acupuncture has been a mainstay of medicine throughout Asia where it is used to maintain health as well as treat disease. It originated during the Han Dynasty in China and was introduced in Europe in the 17th century. Most Americans first heard of acupuncture after President Nixon's 1972 visit to China. Reporters brought back amazing stories of acupuncture's pain-killing properties, including reports of major surgery performed with acupuncture as the only anesthetic.

A key component of traditional Chinese medicine (see page 33), acupuncture is based on the theory that an essential life energy called qi (pronounced chee) flows through the body along invisible channels called meridians that touch every organ. Illness can unbalance your qi, and likewise, out-of-balance qi can cause illness or pain. Stimulation of specific points along the meridians can correct the flow of qi to optimize health, or block pain.

More than 300 major acupuncture points lie along these meridians, and there are several different ways to stimulate them. The most familiar to the West is needle acupuncture, in which very fine metal needles are inserted into the skin at the "acupoints" to manipulate qi. Sometimes, the needles are hooked to a low-level electrical current (electroacupuncture) for a more powerful effect.

Other types of acupuncture stimulate the energy points with heat and herbs (called moxibustion), magnets, low-frequency lasers, or even bee stings. Sometimes larger areas around the points may be treated with "cupping": Small glass cups are heated and put on the skin, forming vacuums as they cool that stimulate the areas under the cups. A practitioner might use more than one of these stimulation types in a treatment.

If the idea of being needled doesn't appeal to you, you can get some of the same benefits from acupressure, an even older form of this therapy. Practitioners stimulate these same points, but instead of needles they use their fingers or tools to apply pressure.

Acupuncture is a puzzlement to many. The invisible channels of qi bear no relationship to

Western understanding of anatomy. Science cannot explain why sticking a needle in your earlobe might relieve the pain in your knee – or why some people respond to acupuncture whereas others do not.

Acupuncture has very real effects, even if we don't quite understand how or why. Brain imaging techniques and other tests have shown that stimulating acupuncture points can cause biologic responses. These responses can affect the blood and immune systems, and can spur the release of chemicals in your muscles, spinal cord and brain that block pain and reduce inflammation (NIH panel report).

Western science can explain some of these effects, at least in relation to pain. The current explanation is that stimulating acupuncture points in turn stimulates the nervous system to release the body's natural pain-killing endorphins and other neurotransmitters that carry messages between nerve cells. These chemicals then either change the experience of pain or trigger the release of other chemicals and hormones that influence the body's internal regulating system.

What Happens in an Acupuncture Treatment

Acupuncture treatments are given in a room that can be as ordinary as your family doctor's office, or in a more gently lighted room smelling of herbs and decorated with Chinese anatomy charts.

A first session typically lasts about an hour and a half, with follow-up sessions taking 30 minutes to an hour. You'll be asked to lie or sit on a padded table, and to remove or loosen just enough clothing to get comfortable and to uncover areas to be treated.

A traditional Chinese medicine practitioner may take a detailed health history, asking many questions about your diet, sleep and bowel habits. He or she will examine your tongue and take your pulse in several different places. Treatment often includes herbs and advice on lifestyle and diet.

For the acupuncture treatment, your practitioner may use from two to 15 hair-thin, sterile disposable needles, either alone or combined with heat or a gentle electric stimulation. They are inserted at specific points that relate to your condition in Chinese medicine, but not necessarily in the area that's bothering you: Neck or back pain, for example, may be treated by stimulating points in your feet.

As the practitioner inserts the very fine needles, you may not even feel them, or you may feel a "pinch," sting and some warmth or tingling. Most people say this doesn't hurt, or hurts only for a few seconds. Practitioners say they can feel the qi respond when they insert needles in the correct spots.

The practitioner may also use his or her hands or a hand-held tool to press on the acupoints (see What Happens in an Acupressure Session). Sometimes tiny amounts of an herb called mugwort (or moxa in China) are burned over the stimulation points. Some practitioners may use a mild electric current with the needles (electroacupuncture); and some use bee stings or venom injections on acupoints.

The acupuncturist will leave you resting with the needles in place anywhere from a few minutes to an hour (20 minutes is typical), checking periodically to make sure you are comfortable or to manipulate or remove some needles. You may be asked to change position after a bit, so needles can be inserted in different acupoints. After the needles are removed, you'll be asked to rest quietly for awhile and then get up slowly, noticing any changes. You may feel a bit lightheaded.

Responses to acupuncture vary widely, even among people with the same disease or symptoms. Some feel an immediate and strong effect, such as an almost-electric tingling or heat, whereas others may not notice anything for several sessions. Your symptoms might disappear completely after a session, or may be worse for a day or so and then improve.

Acupuncturists say acute conditions, such as a sprain or a backache, usually respond within a few sessions. Chronic or long-term conditions, such as the pain associated with many kinds of arthritis, may take one or two treatments a week for several months before the qi is re-balanced. Then you may need follow-up treatments every few months to maintain the balance.

If you show no improvement after several sessions, it may be that acupuncture doesn't work for you. Or you might want to try a different acupuncture technique or a different therapist.

What Happens in an Acupressure Treatment

An acupressure treatment is much the same as acupuncture, but the effect may not be as specific or as powerful. It stimulates the same points, but without the needles and without breaking the skin.

The several types of acupressure use the same or similar points as acupuncture, but they use different techniques. Shiatsu is a Japanese method based on traditional Chinese medicine, see pages 33 and 122. Some methods focus only on pressure points, whereas others include stroking or rubbing motions such as those used in massage, but without using lotions or oils.

For most treatments, you lie on a padded table or a mat on the floor, wearing loose clothing. The practitioner presses on the acupoints, using varying amounts of pressure and holding the points for different amounts of time, from a few seconds to a few minutes. He or she may use the whole hand, fingers, thumbs, elbows and even the feet to press acupoints. Sometimes, the practitioner will use tools such as rollers, balls or pointers to apply pressure.

Do-It-Yourself Acupressure

If acupressure works for you, you can learn to use many of these pressure techniques yourself, anytime and anywhere.

Try pressing on a general pain-relief spot near the base of your thumb to relieve arthritis aches in your hands, arms, neck or shoulders. To find this spot, use your opposite thumb to press the webbing between the thumb and index finger. Feel for a tender spot over toward the base of the index finger bone, and hold for several seconds.

Knee pain can be helped by pressing the center of the bottom of both feet, or a spot on the outside of your calf four finger-widths below the knee (see illustrations).

Of course, you won't be able to reach some spots by yourself, but a family member or friend can help you. Tools and techniques for self-acupressure are available from several sources, and there are books, videos and audio tapes to help you find the points (see Resources). You can also find workshops on acupressure, perhaps at a hospital or health center.

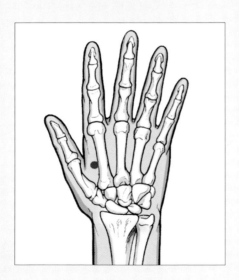
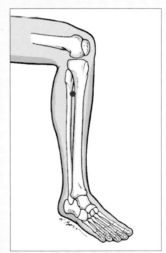

As with acupuncture, not everyone responds to acupressure, and the effects may not be long-lasting. If it doesn't seem to help, you may want to try acupuncture.

Scientific Evidence

The effects of acupuncture use have been documented in thousands of published papers. Many of these studies don't meet scientific standards, or are not published in English. But the evidence overall suggests that acupuncture can ease pain and some other symptoms of arthritis and related diseases.

Since 1980, acupuncture has been endorsed by the World Health Organization for the treatment of some 40 ailments, including osteoarthritis and rheumatoid arthritis. It got a major stamp of approval in 1997 when a National Institutes of Health panel endorsed it for postoperative pain and nausea, and also concluded acupuncture could help in the treatment of fibromyalgia and other musculoskeletal conditions without the side effects of steroid injections or NSAIDs.

Several studies indicate acupuncture can ease the pain of osteoarthritis. One controlled study looked at osteoarthritis of the knee in patients awaiting surgery. The acupuncture group showed a significant reduction in pain and other symptoms compared to the control group. In fact, one-fourth of the patients improved so much, they canceled their scheduled surgeries (Christensen). An uncontrolled study that also looked at acupuncture effects in osteoarthritis of the knee found significant improvement in pain and function at the end of a 12-week treatment (Berman).

An analysis of nine published studies for back pain found acupuncture better than other treatments (Ernst), and two studies showed it is effective for fibromyaliga. In a randomized controlled trial of 70 people with fibromyalgia, electroacupuncture was given to one group while the other received a sham treatment. The treated group had a significant improvement (DeLuze). An uncontrolled study of 29 people with fibromyalgia showed acupuncture treatment resulted in decreased pain levels and fewer tender points (Sprott).

Other randomized, controlled research shows acupuncture eased depression (Allen), and significantly decreased the number and severity of attacks in Raynaud's phenomenon (Appiah). An uncontrolled pilot study showed it helped patients with irritable bowel syndrome (Chan).

However, in a randomized, controlled study of people with Sjögren's syndrome, acupuncture didn't help the treated group (List). Electoacupuncture had no significantly different effect than a sham treatment on a study of those with psoriasis (Jerner). A 1997 analysis of 17 studies looked at acupuncture in inflammatory diseases such as rheumatoid arthritis, spondyloarthropathy, lupus and systemic sclerosis. The authors found the studies failed to show the effectiveness of acupuncture (Lautenschlager).

Acupuncture also was no better than placebo in a British randomized, placebo-controlled study of 56 patients with rheumatoid arthritis (David). Only single-point acupuncture was used in the study, however.

There are fewer available acupressure studies, and most deal with controlling nausea. However, because acupressure stimulates the same acupoints as acupuncture, it may have similar effects. One uncontrolled study found do-it-yourself acupressure for tension and migraine headaches as effective as prescription drugs (Kurland).

Expert Opinion

Acupuncture is an accepted treatment in many parts of the world for arthritis and related conditions. While its effectiveness has not been definitively proven, there's enough research to suggest it can help control pain, and that it is safe when performed by a trained professional using sterile disposable needles. Acupressure, which doesn't break the skin, is even safer but lacks evidence of effectiveness.

These techniques are probably worth a try, especially if other treatments aren't working for you. They may be helpful supplements to your regular medical regimen. If you are taking NSAIDs for pain, but not for inflammation, you may get enough relief from acupuncture to reduce your dosage – and the potential NSAID side effects. However, you may need regular acupuncture treatments to keep that benefit. Because acupuncture may not be covered by your insurance you'll need to weigh the cost of acupuncture treatments against the possible side effects of long-term NSAID use.

Most importantly, don't abandon treatments prescribed by your doctor. A reputable acupuncturist will urge you to work with your medical doctor, and will be willing to talk with your doctor about your treatment.

Finding a Therapist
Acupuncture

There are an estimated 10,000 acupuncturists in the United States. Many – but not all – states require licensing. Some states license acupuncture alone, others include other forms of Oriental medicine such as herbs and manual therapies such as massage.

The major certifying board for acupuncturists is the National Certification Commission for Acupuncture and Oriental Medicine (NCCAOM). It has certified about 9,000 practitioners who have met national professional standards.

If you prefer a medical doctor, the American Academy of Medical Acupuncture has a membership of about 1,400 medical doctors and doctors of osteopathy who have completed 220 hours of training in acupuncture. Overall, about 4,000 doctors have some kind of acupuncture

Organizations

National Certification Commission for Acupuncture and Oriental Medicine
11 Canal Center Plaza, Suite 330
Alexandria, VA 22314
Phone: 703/548-9004
Web site: http://www.nccaom.org/
Certifies acupuncturists and has a directory of practitioners.

The American Institute of Oriental Medicine
433 Front Street
Catasauqua, PA 18032
Phone: 610/266-1433
E-mail: aaoml@aol.com
Web site: http://www.aaom.com
Has a referral list.

National Acupuncture and Oriental Medicine Alliance
14637 Starr Road, SE
Olalla, WA 98359
Phone: 253/851-6896
Web site: http://www.acuall.org
Provides referrals for acupuncturists and information on insurance coverage, state and other legislation that involves acupuncture.

The American Academy of Medical Acupuncture
5820 Wilshire Boulevard, Suite 500
Los Angeles, CA 90036
Phone: 800/521-2262 or 323/937-5514
Web site: http://www.medicalacupuncture.org
Membership is limited to medical doctors and doctors of osteopathy who have completed a training program of 220 hours. It maintains a directory of practitioners, and its Web site has good basic information and links to other useful sites.

NIH Consensus Program Information Center
P.O. Box 2577
Kensington, MD 20891
Phone: 888/644-2667
Web site: http://odp.od.nih.gov/consensus/cons/107/107_intro.htm
Has available the NIH Consensus Development Statement on Acupuncture.

The Acupressure Institute
1533 Shattuck Avenue
Berkeley, CA 94709
Phone: 800/442-2232 or 510/845-1059
Web site: http://www.205.180.191.2/acupressure
Has information and a catalog of products.

Books

Arthritis Relief at Your Fingertips, by Michael Reed Gach. 1989. New York. Time Warner. Paperback. $15.99. An illustrated guide to acupressure techniques.

Between Heaven and Earth: A Guide to Chinese Medicine, by Harriet Beinfield and Efrem Korngold. 1992. New York. Ballantine Books. $14.

The Web That Has No Weaver: Understanding Chinese Medicine, by Ted J. Kaptchuk. 1983. Lincolnwood, IL. NTC Publishing Group. Paperback. $11.95.

Audio Tape
Arthritis Relief at your Fingertips: Morning & Evening Routines, Michael Reed Gach. Order from Enhanced Audio Systems by writing 190 Powell St, Suite 1135, Emeryville, CA 94608 or by calling 415/652-4009.

Web Sites
Acupuncture.com has many informative links.
http://www.acupuncture.com/AcuPoints/acupuncture.html

The Qi Journal
This informative Web site has articles on many forms of holistic medicine, a product catalog, and an interactive acupuncture model.
http://www.qi-journal.com

training, and treatments from them are more likely to be covered by your health insurance. However, a medical degree isn't a guarantee of expertise in acupuncture. Be sure the doctor has completed a recognized acupuncture training program. It takes years to master the theory and technique, and traditional Chinese medicine acupuncturists say many doctors who take up acupuncture don't have adequate training. They recommend finding a therapist who has many years of experience and who is trained in traditional Chinese medicine.

Contact one of the national certification boards or agencies for a directory of practitioners (see Resources).

Acupressure
It's not known how many acupressurists are practicing in the United States because they are not necessarily certified through a national board and are not required to be licensed. Some are certified through the NCCAOM. In some states, they are required to be licensed as massage therapists and many massage therapists use acupressure techniques. Ask if the practitioner has a certificate from an acupressure school.

Self-help acupressure techniques are taught through some health providers, or at community and senior centers. Workshops are often advertised in new-age publications. If you can't find a practitioner, you might consult a book that shows where and how to apply pressure for your complaint. Some specialized bookstores, catalogs or Web sites also sell videos (see Resources).

Cautions

! Be sure the acupuncture practitioner uses sterile disposable needles.

! Be sure to tell the practitioner about all health conditions, including pregnancy; and to list all medications you are taking, especially blood-thinners, glucocorticoids and anti-seizure medications.

! Acupuncture isn't generally recommended for children 8 years old or younger, because they have trouble remaining still long enough for a treatment.

Good Advice

• Be sure the acupuncture practitioner is certified or licensed, and that the acupressure practitioner meets requirements in your state for massage therapists.

• Ask how many sessions your condition requires. If you don't seem to improve after four to six sessions, this therapy may not work for you. Or you may want to try another therapist.

• Take it easy for several hours before and after a treatment: Eat lightly, and don't drink alcohol or engage in sexual activity. Therapists say these activities may interfere with the effects of the treatment. Plan to rest after the treatment to get the most benefit.

• Many practitioners offer herbal remedies, which are generally safe when dispensed by an expert. But remember: Herbs are powerful medicine, and can have unwanted effects or interact with other medications. Be sure the practitioner knows all the prescription and over-the-counter drugs you are taking. Or play it extra safe, and don't take the herbs.

• Keep written notes about your response to the treatment, and tell your doctor and acupuncturist about any changes so that the follow-up treatments and all of your medications can be designed to best help you.

• There are many different styles of acupuncture. Although all use the concept of moving qi, they emphasize different acupuncture points and techniques. So if one style or therapist doesn't seem to work for you, you might want to explore another type or therapist. Discuss this with your acupuncturist.

Costs

Costs vary in different locations. A first acupuncture or acupressure visit may cost between $75 and $150. Follow-up visits cost between $35 and $75. These fees may include herbs. Some health insurers will cover these treatments, especially if prescribed by – or performed by – a doctor.

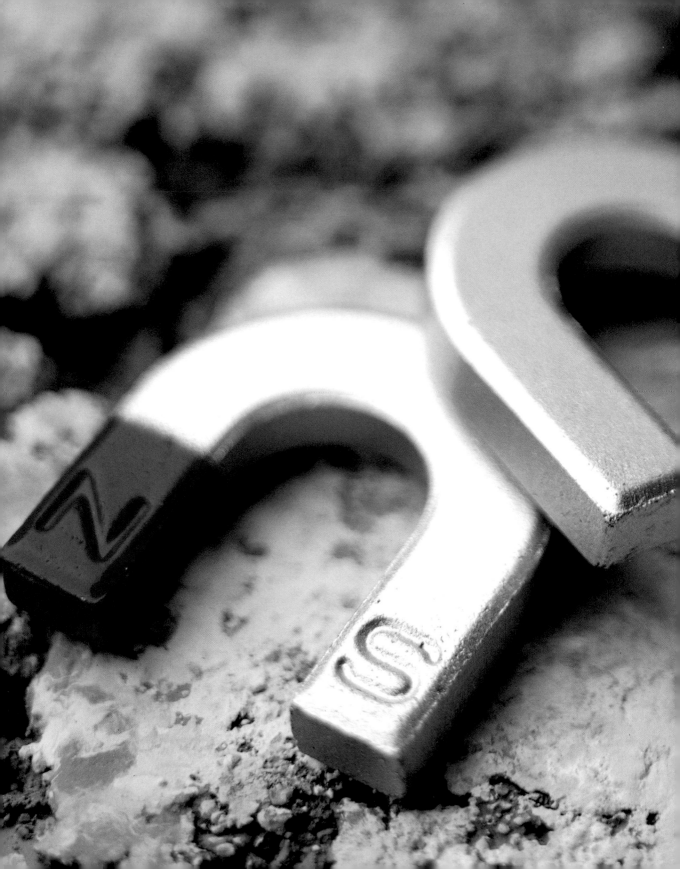

Miscellaneous Therapies

BEES, BRACELETS, LASERS AND MAGNETS

There are many complementary therapies for arthritis that don't seem to fall into any one category. Here's a review of some of the better-known therapies.

BEE VENOM THERAPY

Most of us go out of the way to avoid bee stings. But some are willing to endure hundreds or even thousands of stings or injections of bee venom, claiming it helps their arthritis and other musculoskeletal ills. Some say several sessions of stings relieve their symptoms completely, others return for "booster" sessions every few months.

Bee sting therapy is widely used in Asia, Eastern Europe and the former Soviet Union. In the United States, it's more of an underground therapy popularized by word-of-mouth and beekeepers. In fact, there's a society of beekeepers who support and offer this therapy, and businesses that sell live bees by mail for sting therapy (see Resources).

How It's Used

Bee stings or injections are usually done on or near the painful areas. They might also be given on trigger points for pain, or at acupoints (the points selected for acupuncture treatments).

The venom can be given via "nature's hypodermic" from live bees, or by injections of purified bee venom. Injections, which are usually given by doctors, have the advantage of medical help being nearby if you have an allergic reaction. However, bee experts say these shots don't contain the whole, fresh venom and thus are not as effective as being stung by a live bee.

For treatment with live bee stings, the bee is usually grasped with a pair of long tweezers and placed on the spot to be stung. The stings can be very painful, and you may need many stings or injections to see any effect. To lessen the pain, the area to be treated is often iced before and after the process. (The process usually kills the bees, by the way.) If you don't see any improvement after about eight sessions and a total of 20–70 stings or injections, it probably won't work for you. Some practitioners suggest a longer trial. If you decide to go the real bee route, find a beekeeper or other expert experienced in this therapy to help you.

RESORCES *
BEE VENOM THERAPY

Organization
American Apitherapy Society
Linda Day, Office Coordinator
5370 Carmel Road
Hillsboro, OH 45133
Phone: 937/466-9214
E-mail: lday@in-touch.net
Web site: http://www.apitherapy.org
This organization promotes medicinal uses of bee products, and has information about how to safely perform bee sting therapy. It will also supply names of members you can talk to about bee therapies.

Book
Health and the Honeybee, by Charles Mraz. 1995. Queen City Publications. Paperback. $12.95. This book is by beekeeper Mraz, who is in his 90s and has been offering apitherapy for 60 years.

Scientific Evidence

There may be something to bee sting therapy: Analysis shows bee venom contains powerful anti-inflammatories and other chemicals that can reduce pain. In animal studies, venom relieved inflammation (Chang), and it appeared to prevent rats from getting an induced arthritis (Eiseman, Zurier). But there aren't any studies on humans, and venom can provoke a sometimes-fatal allergic reaction.

Expert Opinion

There are thousands of anecdotal reports of bee stings relieving the symptoms of arthritis. But because there aren't any human clinical trials that show bee venom helps arthritis or any other ailment, most doctors say it's not worth the risk (see Cautions). Also, it's such an unpleasant, painful and potentially dangerous therapy that even doctors who use it say it's a last resort, when nothing else seems to control pain or other symptoms.

Finding a Practitioner

Purified bee venom is available, but bee venom injections are FDA-approved only to help desensitize people to bee allergies. Thus few physicians give bee venom injections for any other reason. Those who do may not charge for the venom, because it is not an approved procedure. Your best bet for finding a physician to give injections is probably word-of-mouth. Some chronic pain clinics may be able to give you a reference as well.

Beekeepers, however, often help people get live bee stings. You can find a beekeeper in your area through the American Apitherapy Society (see Resources). Several beekeepers and bee sting proponents also have Web sites. You can order live bees for do-it-yourself stings, but experts advise first learning the procedure from someone experienced in bee sting therapy.

Cautions

! Some people develop an allergic reaction to bee venom: A severe reaction, called anaphylactic shock, can be fatal. Most allergic reactions to stinging insects are to wasps and yellow jackets rather than honeybees.

! You (and anyone else who will be around when using live bees) should be tested for bee venom allergy before beginning treatment. However, anyone might suddenly develop an allergic reaction at any time, even those who have been stung many times before.

! Never sting yourself when alone. Always have an emergency sting kit with you, and know the number and location of the nearest emergency facility.

! Ask your doctor for a prescription for a sting kit, which contains epinephrine; and make sure you have no contraindication for self-administered epinephrine. You will need to go immediately to an emergency facility if you have a reaction, and if you use the kit because epinephrine can have severe side effects.

Costs

Beekeepers will often help you with – or give – bee stings for free. Purchasing bees by mail costs about $10 for 60 live bees, plus shipping. Injections of bee venom extract by your physician may be covered by insurance as an office visit.

COPPER BRACELETS

Folklore has it that wearing copper bracelets eases arthritis pain. A placebo-controlled study of 300 people that compared copper bracelets to bracelets painted to look like copper had surprising results. A significant number of those wearing copper said they got some relief. The copper bracelets lost weight in the process, which theoretically could be from absorption into the body of the wearer (Walker).

Scientific Evidence

It is possible to have a copper deficiency, but a recommended daily intake has not been established. At any rate, it's doubtful you're getting any copper from wearing a bracelet. For one thing, if it stays shiny, it's probably lacquered to prevent tarnishing – and that also prevents the copper from contacting your skin. Some are skeptical that copper is absorbed through the skin anyway.

Expert Opinion

Wearing a copper bracelet won't hurt, but there's not enough scientific evidence that it helps.

Finding a Bracelet

These products are sold in new-age stores, through catalogs and through online suppliers on the Internet.

Good Advice

- If you decide to buy a copper bracelet, get an inexpensive one that hasn't been treated to prevent tarnishing, so the copper will be in touch with your skin.

Costs

Like any jewelry, prices will vary, ranging from $7–$15 or so. There are also copper rings and discs that stick on the back of your watch.

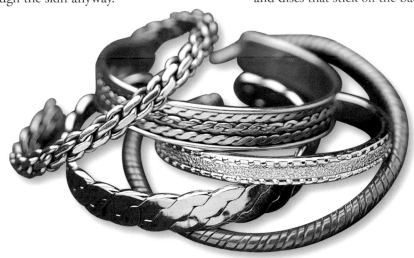

LOW ENERGY LASER THERAPY

Lasers, which use the magic of light, have become important tools in medicine. They have made possible many delicate procedures by allowing surgeons to cut, burn or coagulate tissue with extreme precision.

There is another, completely different, kind of laser called low energy laser light (LELL) that's used for soft tissue injuries. Sometimes called cold laser, it emits a much gentler energy that can penetrate deep into tissues without damaging them. Proponents say this deep light stimulates cell repair, increases circulation and relieves inflammation and pain. One theory is that the deep light changes the chemical balance in cells, and that it may also stimulate production of neurotransmitters (the chemicals that carry information among cells).

Low energy laser light therapy has been around since 1979 and is approved for use in many other countries, but not the United States. It is used for various musculoskeletal conditions, including osteoarthritis and rheumatoid arthritis, fibromyalgia, carpal tunnel syndrome, sprains, strains and soft tissue injuries. The treatment takes about five minutes, and a series of 15 sessions is usual for most chronic conditions. The effects can last for a year: Some say it lasts much longer, but others come for regular maintenance treatments.

How It's Used

The LELL tool looks rather like a flashlight from the outside. A physical therapist or physician gives the treatments, in which the instrument is put right against the skin at a trigger point, hot spot or painful point.

Scientific Evidence

Treatment with LELL is not FDA-approved for use in the United States except as an investigational therapy. Manufacturers of the instrument say it is undergoing clinical trials here now.

Although laser therapy is widely used in other countries, there are few acceptable published human studies that show it is effective. A Dutch review looked at 36 randomized clinical trials of the effects of LELL on 1,704 patients with various musculoskeletal and skin disorders. Although the overall results were better than placebo, and significantly better for those with rheumatoid arthritis, the studies were poorly done so no definite conclusions could be reached (Beckerman). In an uncontrolled U.S. study, seven to 15 treatments reversed carpal tunnel syndrome in 77 percent of the 30 people treated (Weintraub 1). But four other double-blind, placebo-controlled studies of laser therapy for OA (Bulow) or RA (Hall, Heussler, Johannsen) found no clinically relevant effects.

Expert Opinion

Laser therapy is widely used, including on animals. But the reports are mixed. Some doctors say this works, others say it's a placebo effect. Either way, it's only approved for investigational use in the United States and is not easily available.

Finding a Practitioner

Low energy laser light therapy is not approved for use in the United States unless you are part of the ongoing clinical trials. It's just not known when – or if – LELL will be approved for use in the United States.

However, it is available in other countries. Ask your doctor for advice on finding a reputable clinic, or contact a researcher listed in the studies we cite in the appendix. We found a number of Web sites from manufacturers, but decided not to list them here because we were not able to verify the quality of their instruments or clinics.

Cautions

! Distributors of LELL devices claim the therapy has no adverse side effects.

! There is a possibility of irreversible eye damage from staring directly into the instrument, so protective eyewear is used during treatments.

! Because results are not known for several conditions, LELL therapy is not recommended for cancer, pregnancy or diabetic neuropathy.

Costs

The LELL tool costs about $9,000. A treatment costs the equivalent of $30–$50, or more and is usually not covered by insurance. (Treatments for those enrolled in clinical trials are usually done at no charge to the patient.)

MAGNET THERAPY

Magnets hold a big attraction for those in pain. Permanent magnets similar to those used to hold notes and photos on your refrigerator door are being marketed as a treatment for the pains of osteoarthritis, fibromyalgia and many other conditions. They are a favorite with athletes, and have become a $1.5-billion-dollar-a-year business.

The magnets come in all shapes and sizes. They can be ordered in thin strips or discs that attach directly to the body (like *Band-Aids*), or snuggled into braces, splints and wraps. Also available are magnet-studded facial masks, car seats, mattress pads, shoe insoles and collars for your pets.

Claims that magnets help healing go back for centuries. History has it that Cleopatra slept with a magnetic lode-stone to prevent aging, and Franz Anton Mesmer, who plied his magic magnet trade in the late 1700s, is probably the most famous – and infamous – magnet therapist. In various forms, magnet therapies were popular until the advent of antibiotics around World War II.

No one knows how magnets are supposed to work to relieve pain (or if indeed they do), but there are some theories. The idea is that electricity is everywhere – including in our bodies – and that putting magnets on sore spots could increase circulation, suppress inflammation, affect C-fibers that transmit pain, change the polarization of cells – or all of the above.

Magnets come in different strengths, which is measured in gauss. The strength of the earth's natural magnetic field is about 0.05 gauss; refrigerator magnets are about 60 gauss, and the magnets being sold for therapy range from about 300 to 4,000 gauss.

How They Are Used

Magnets often come with wraps or bandages to hold them in place. You put them on your body over the area that aches, or use the magnet-studded shoe insoles, car seat covers and mattress pads. Some experts think the wraps the magnets come in make sore joints feel better by supporting and warming them.

Scientific Evidence

So far, there is little evidence to support claims that magnets could ease arthritis symptoms. There are two independent and scientifically accepted trials on humans, and one on animals. In the animal study, rats with inflamed joints that spent three weeks in a cage magnetized to 3,800 gauss showed a significant decrease in inflammation levels (Weinberger).

Although this is intriguing, few of us would want to spend all of our time in a magnetic field – even supposing it would be practical to create and maintain one large enough.

A double-blind, placebo-controlled study of static magnets on post-polio pain got a lot of press a few years ago. It compared magnets to fake magnets designed to look the same. Results showed 76 percent of those who placed a magnet on a sore spot for 45 minutes said their pain was decreased, whereas only 19 percent of those with the fake magnets felt any improvement (Vallbona). However, the study consisted of one treatment per patient and didn't say how long the pain relief lasted.

A more recent study gave magnetized shoe insoles to 19 people with peripheral neuropathy of the feet, a painful condition caused by poor circulation. In the randomized, double-blind, placebo-controlled trial, nine of the 10 participants whose condition was caused by diabetes reported significantly less pain. Of those with non-diabetic peripheral neuropathy, three of 10 reported pain relief (Weintraub 2).

Expert Opinion

Magnet therapy holds promise, but needs more research. Most experts say the low-level static magnets being sold are a waste of money. Meanwhile, be wary of magnet marketers: Many magnet marketers falsely claim there is accepted scientific proof magnets can help osteoarthritis. This is not true. They may be referring to studies of electromagnetic therapy, where a pulsed electric current is passed through a permanent magnet. This is a medically accepted therapy and a completely different procedure (see PEMF on page 156). Some vendors claim their static magnets have special designs that make them more effective, but there's no evidence to support this.

However, some people say these magnets help ease their pain. If you want to try it, most doctors have no objection. Start with a small investment and ask for a money-back guarantee before you buy.

Cautions

! The biggest risk seems to be to your pocketbook, but magnets may affect your electronic instruments.

! Don't use magnets if you have a pacemaker or other surgically implanted electronic device that could be affected. Check with your doctor first.

! Magnet-sensitive electronics such as switches on electric heating blankets could be affected, causing injuries.

! If permanent magnets do work as claimed – that is, increase circulation – they could cause some medications to be absorbed more quickly. As always, keep note of any changes while you are using them.

Good Advice

- Static magnets are probably harmless for most people as long as you don't use them to replace your regular therapies.

Costs

Small patches start at less than $5; prices go up to $1,000 or more for king-size mattress pads.

PULSED ELECTROMAGNETIC THERAPY

There is a magnet treatment that is medically accepted for some uses, and studies have shown it may work for osteoarthritis. It's called pulsed electromagnetic field therapy (PEMF) and it's been used successfully for more than a decade to stimulate the healing of broken bones. It's approved for other uses in more than 20 countries and is widely used in Europe for OA and other musculoskeletal conditions.

PEMF is not approved for use in the United States. It's being investigated at several major universities, and studies have shown it can relieve the pain of OA of the knee and spine. It's painless, noninvasive and has no reported side effects. But it's not cheap and is not likely to be covered by insurance.

The theory is that PEMF stimulates repair by replacing a short circuit in the normal electrical process in our bodies. It's known that bones and other parts of our bodies produce electrical signals. It is believed that under normal circumstances tiny electrical currents set off when we move or walk stimulate bone and cartilage growth. Bone or joint damage, such as cartilage loss in OA, can interrupt that stimulation. Low-level doses of external electrical stimulation may signal the body to repair cartilage.

What Happens in a Session

This isn't a do-it-yourself proposition. You have to go to a place that has the machines to create this pulsed magnetic field. In the treatments, you place the sore body part inside a circular magnetic coil device that looks like a doughnut. Low-level electric currents are run through the coils, creating an electromagnetic field through which a pulsed signal is sent to the area being treated. The treatments are painless.

Scientific Evidence

So far, there is no proof that PEMF can grow new cartilage. But studies do show it relieves pain and improves function. Two

RESOURCE ✳ PEMF

Company
Pulsed Signal Therapy
881 Alma Real Drive, Suite 301
Pacific Palisades, CA 90272
Phone: 888/459-2100
E-mail: info@certifiedpst.com
Web site: http://www.certifiedpst.com
or http://www.pstworld.com
Provides information on treatment
centers in other countries.

studies were done at Yale University using an electromagnetic coil device. The first, a double-blind, placebo-controlled pilot study involving 18 people with OA of the knee, showed that those who got 18 half-hour treatments had an average improvement of 23 to 61 percent in pain, joint tenderness and discomfort. The placebo group that got fake treatments had two to 18 percent improvement (Trock 1). A later Yale study with 167 patients with OA of the knee or cervical spine showed similar, significant improvements (Trock 2).

Another double-blind, placebo-controlled study was also done at Johns Hopkins University where 78 patients with OA of the knee had four weeks of treatments or a placebo. The treated group had significantly better results in terms of pain, function and physician assessment than the placebo group (Zizic).

PEMF is also being promoted for carpal tunnel syndrome and for rheumatoid arthritis, but so far there are no studies that show it helps these conditions.

Expert Opinion

PEMF therapy looks promising and appears to have no side effects. It might be worth a try, if you can afford it – and the time to travel to get it. At the time of publication, it wasn't approved in the United States but is available in more than 100 clinics in other countries.

Finding a Practitioner

A United States company, Pulsed Signal Therapy, provides therapy at clinics in Tijuana, Mexico, and Vancouver, B.C. The treatments are also available in Europe, the Bahamas and other vacation spots.

Cautions

! PEMF therapy is not advisable for anyone who is pregnant or who has cancer because it may affect cell growth.

! Consult with your doctor if you have a pacemaker.

Costs

A session of nine one-hour treatments over a five-day period costs about $1,800. This does not include travel, hotel or other expenses, and treatments are not covered by insurance.

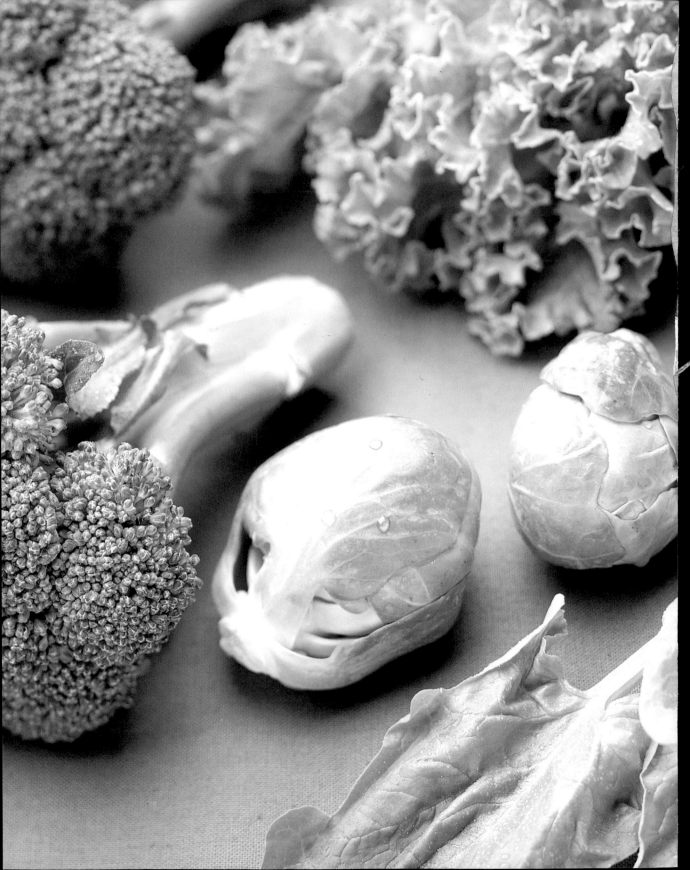

Food and Arthritis

THE DIET CONNECTION

Special diets have been connected with healing and with spiritual and religious practices since antiquity. For just about as long, diet has been suspected as a prime cause of arthritis. All kinds of "arthritis diets" have been proposed, and bookstores today are crowded with cookbooks, diet books and health books that promise to cure arthritis and whatever else ails you. Little of this information is based on science, and quite a bit of it is wrong. With the exception of gout (see page 169), there is no clear-cut proof that what you eat can either cause or cure the many kinds of arthritis and musculoskeletal disorders.

So until recently, most rheumatologists regarded diet therapy for arthritis as pure quackery. Now, as scientists learn more about the connection between diet and disease, they are taking another look. Diet affects your overall health, and what we eat has been shown to play a role in many disorders, including heart disease, stroke, and colon and breast cancer.

There is growing evidence that changing your diet may help ease some symptoms and possibly even influence the progression of rheumatoid arthritis (Darlington 1). In fact, food may be a new frontier in managing chronic ailments and preventing disease, as scientists learn more about the complex effects of nutrition.

There is still much research to be done, but scientists believe there are several ways in which diet might affect your arthritis.

- A small number of people with arthritis and related musculoskeletal disorders might be sensitive to certain foods that could trigger symptoms, or worsen them.

- A diet high in certain foods – such as saturated animal fats and the most commonly used vegetable oils – can affect the complex inflammatory response, and they could contribute to joint and tissue inflammation.

- Diet can make your general health worse, or affect other diseases you may have such as diabetes or heart disease, which in turn can affect how your body handles the arthritis symptoms.

- Arthritis can make your diet worse. It can keep you from getting good nutrition, because aching joints make it difficult to shop for and prepare food, and may even cause problems with chewing and eating. Pain and fatigue can ruin your appetite.

Checking for Food Sensitivities

If you use common sense, you can safely try cutting out one specific food at a time, starting with the most common offenders, and see if it seems to help. Start keeping a food diary by writing down everything you eat and drink, and any change in symptoms. After a month, you may have an idea of a food that could be provoking symptoms. (Do remember that arthritis can have remissions and flares that are not connected with foods or anything else.) You can try eliminating that one food from your diet for two weeks to see what happens. At the end of two weeks, begin eating the food again to see if there are any changes in your symptoms.

Don't cut out a whole food category, such as all vegetables or all fruits – just try one food at a time. Use common sense: If you are going to cut out dairy, for example, be sure you get the needed calcium and vitamin D from a supplement or other food. Don't do this for more than two weeks, and be sure to tell your doctor what you are doing.

If you think you have identified a symptom-producing food, see an allergist and a dietitian before you make a decision to cut it out of your diet forever. Get a good diet plan for your individual situation.

However, there is no actual "arthritis diet" because there are so many kinds of arthritis. Until research proves a definite connection between a specific food and a type of arthritis, your best bet is to eat the kind of diet that's recommended by the American Heart Association or the American Cancer Society. These diets are low in saturated fats and calories, and rich with fruits, vegetables and grains. Watching the types of oils and fats you eat may also help (see Balancing Fats in Your Diet, page 170).

Eating wisely is kind to your whole body, and can cut your risks for many diseases. It can stabilize your weight, helping those who are overweight to take off some of those joint-crushing pounds. Because eating wisely may make you feel better, it may make it easier for those who have lost weight from RA, lupus or fibromyalgia to enjoy food more and add back some pounds.

THE FACTS ABOUT ARTHRITIS DIETS

There must be a book published every week that promises to cure what ails you with a "special" diet. Or you may hear about a "health" diet from a friend or family member. Often these diets give bad nutritional advice that can make your arthritis worse, or cause another medical problem.

Sometimes these diets do contain bits of good advice, but put it to bad use. An example is the so-called Zen or macrobiotic diet that is based on a vegetarian diet, but takes it to extremes. The basic macrobiotic diet is restrictive, but if planned carefully can meet your nutritional needs. As a person progresses to "higher" levels of the diet plan, however, more and more foods are cut out. This can cause serious malnutrition. In children, such a limited diet can retard growth and mental development. Other fad diets are based on certain food combinations, or on apple cider, wheat germ, alfalfa, molasses and so on as a "cure."

When considering a diet, do a little research. And remember: A doctor's name on a diet doesn't mean it's effective or good for you.

Here's a look at some diet strategies, and what researchers have to say about them.

Food Allergies and Sensitivities

It's always tempting to try to pin the cause of a chronic disease on one factor, such as food allergies or sensitivities. Unfortunately, it's not that simple. Although many people think they are allergic or sensitive to certain foods, true food allergies are pretty rare.

For this reason, doctors have dismissed the food sensitivity theory as a cause of arthritis. But now some aren't so sure. So many people report changes in symptoms when they eat or stop eating certain foods that it's worth investigating.

Scientific Evidence

A few studies have shown eliminating certain foods relieved symptoms for some people (Darlington 2, van de Laar, Panush 1). A wide range of foods has been connected with rheumatoid arthritis flares, and there's no consistency. Some people who react to one or two, don't react to any of the others. Among the many suspect foods are dairy products, wheat, corn, beef, pork, peanuts, coffee, eggs and food from the "nightshade" family such as potatoes and tomatoes. Some people also find that some food additives or seasonings – such as salt, MSG and nitrates in bacon and lunchmeats – make them feel worse.

Researchers do know that red meat and the most commonly used vegetable oils (such as corn, sunflower and safflower oils) break down into arachidonic acids, which are building

Recognizing a Fad Diet

Beware of diets that can harm. Here are some questions to ask yourself about the latest "arthritis diet."

- Does it stress one food or only a few foods, and ask you to eliminate all others? Such diets will often have names such as "the grapefruit diet."

- Does it claim to cure your arthritis? With the exceptions of gout, bacterial arthritis and Lyme disease, there are no curable forms of arthritis.

- Are its advertisements misleading in that they are made to look like news articles, and not ads?

- Is the sales pitch based on testimonials from people who have been "cured," and not on scientific evidence?

- Does it lack any scientific evidence in the form of published research to back up the claims (see Looking at the Scientific Evidence, page 14)?

- Can there be harmful effects from following the diet?

blocks for the prostaglandins and leukotrienes that cause pain and inflammation. Studies also suggest that some people with arthritis and musculoskeletal disorders have problems with digestion and food absorption. One theory involving the connection between digestion and arthritis and related disorders is "leaky gut" syndrome. The theory holds that some conditions may make the intestines "leaky" and allow food molecules and bacteria to pass through the membrane walls. These misplaced molecules can then provoke or worsen a systemic immune response and inflammation (Bjarnason).

Expert Opinion

So far, most of the studies on food sensitivities are based on anecdotal information, case studies or uncontrolled studies. And autoimmune diseases are known to have flares and remissions, so it's not easy to tell what — if anything — caused a change in symptoms. As research reveals more connections between diet and health, it seems likely that certain foods may turn out to increase symptoms and inflammation for some people. For now, however, there's simply a lack of consistency, so no specific or general recommendations can be given.

Elimination Diets

The purpose of elimination diets is to discover what types of food – if any – might be connected with some of your symptoms. Although you can experiment on your own with eliminating one type of food from your diet, such as dairy products, a true elimination diet is more restrictive and needs supervision by a health professional. The most accurate will be blinded, as in a scientific study, so that you don't know what you are eating (See Looking at the Scientific Evidence, page 14).

It takes months to do a true elimination diet, and it can be hazardous to your health. Elimination diets usually begin with a fast, during which you can only eat or drink a very limited number of foods. Some fasts allow only water or fruit juices (see Fasting). After a three- to 10-day fast to allow your body to cycle-out any food you've eaten, you begin adding foods one at a time to see if there is a reaction. Sometimes elimination diets identify food sensitivities or allergies, such as an allergy to milk (Ratner, Panush 1)

Expert Opinion

If you suspect certain foods might be contributing to flares and other symptoms, get some professional help. A full-blown elimination diet isn't something to do on your own: You already have one disease, don't add malnutrition to it. Get a referral to a gastrointestinal specialist, an allergist or a registered dietitian. Ask these specialists to help you sort through your diet and see if there could be any connections to your arthritis.

Fasting

Fasting has been practiced for thousands of years for spiritual purposes. It is said to clear the body and the mind, and it plays a role in many major religions. It is also used by many health-conscious people, who may practice a limited fast (where they take only juice and water for a day or so). Fasting may be used before beginning an elimination diet, to clear the body of all foods.

Scientific Evidence

Studies show fasting can bring relief to some people with rheumatoid arthritis – sometimes dramatic relief. But it isn't an effective treatment for arthritis because it doesn't last: Controlled studies show that when the fast ended, the symptoms returned or even worsened (Skoldstam 1). Researchers speculate that fasting may relieve symptoms for some with autoimmune diseases because of the caloric deprivation, which suppresses the immune system and the inflammatory response; or because the intestines are less "leaky" then. Relief could

Organizations

American Dietetic Association
216 West Jackson Boulevard
Chicago, IL 60606-6995
Phone: 800/366-1655 for recorded messages and referrals to a registered dietitian or 900/225-5267 to talk to a registered dietitian. There's a charge of $1.95 for the first minute, 95 cents for each additional minute.
Web site: http://www.eatright.org

Food and Drug Administration
Office of Consumer Affairs, HFE-88
Rockville, MD 20857
Food Information Phone Line: 800/FDA-4010
To ask about a product: 800/532-4440
E-mail: execsec@oc.fda.gov
Web site: http://www.fda.gov/opacom/morecons.html

Eat Right Hotline
Phone: 800/231-DIET (3438)
A Nutrition Information Service provided by the University of Alabama at Birmingham.
A registered dietitian will answer questions.

Alabama Tone Your Bone Hotline
Phone: 888/934-BONE (2663)

U.S. Flax Institute
Box 5051, University Station
North Dakota State University
Fargo, ND 58105-5051
Phone: 701/231-7971
E-mail: buringru@plains.nodak.edu
Web site: http://www.ndsu.nodak.edu/instruct/hammond/dept/flaxinst.htm
For flax information, recipes and where to buy flax products.

Books

All About Omega-3 Oils (Frequently Asked Questions), by Jack Challem (Editor). 1999. Avery Publishing Group. $2.99.

Diet and Arthritis, by Gail Darlington, MD, and Linda Gamlin. 1998. Trafalgar Square. Paperback. $17.95.

The Omega Plan: The Life Saving Nutritional Program Based on the Diet of the Island of Crete, by Artemis P. Simopoulos, MD, and Jo Robinson. 1999. New York. Harper Collins. Paperback. $14.

Cookbooks

The Essential Arthritis Cookbook: Kitchen Basics for People with Arthritis, Fibromyalgia and Other Chronic Pain and Fatigue, by Sarah Morgan, MD, and the Arthritis Center at the University of Alabama at Birmingham. 1996. Mankato, Minn. Appletree Press. Hardcover. $24.95.

Help Yourself – Recipes and Resources from the Arthritis Foundation. Nashville, TN: Arthritis Foundation. Spiral Bound. $12.95. Can be ordered by calling 800/207-8633.

The New Soy Cookbook: Delicious Ideas for Soybeans, Soy Milk, Tofu, Tempeh, Miso and Soy Sauce, by Lorna Sass. 1998. San Francisco. Chronicle Books. Paperback. $17.95. Tells you what to do with tofu, tempeh and other meatless proteins recommended by many nutritionists.

Web Sites

Also see organizations.

American Council on Science and Health
http://www.acsh.org

Tufts University Nutrition Navigator
http://navigator.tufts.edu

also be due to removal of foods that, in some people, seem to cause a sensitivity reaction.

Expert Opinion

Obviously, fasting is not a long-term solution. You'll starve to death before you starve your rheumatoid arthritis into remission. In spite of the evidence that it helps some rheumatoid arthritis symptoms temporarily, it's not a good idea for those with chronic illnesses. People with rheumatoid arthritis have less muscle and more fat than people without arthritis, so fasting is more harmful to them because they start out with lower protein reserves. You need to nourish your body carefully with a well-balanced diet. For those with gout, even limited fasting may set off a gout attack. If you want to consider a fast, consult your doctor and a registered dietitian for instructions.

Nightshade-free Diets

Just about anyone with arthritis has heard the theory that foods from the family *Solanaceae*, or nightshade family, cause joint inflammation. These foods include tomatoes, potatoes, eggplants and peppers.

The theory was developed by Norman F. Childers, PhD, a horticulturist, who noticed his diverticulitis (inflammation of a portion of the intestine) and arthritis symptoms seemed to be aggravated by nightshade foods. As a plant expert, he knew that tomatoes were once considered poisonous. He conducted a seven-year uncontrolled study of about 5,000 people with arthritis who were asked to avoid nightshade foods. Nearly three-fourths of these people said their pain and disability improved on the diet (Childers).

Scientific Evidence

There have been no rigorous studies to confirm Childers' theory, but certain rheumatologists say they have seen some patients improve after removing nightshade foods from their diet.

Expert Opinion

It probably won't hurt you to experiment with this diet, but it can be tricky if you eat out a lot – or like pizza, marinara sauce on your pasta, and ketchup. Remember: Eliminating whole groups of foods such as all fruits or all vegetables can be dangerous.

Dairy-free Diets

It's well-known that some people, regardless of whether they have arthritis, don't have the enzyme (lactase) needed to digest the sugar (lactose) in dairy products. These people who are "lactose intolerant" have to avoid diary altogether, or take medication to replace the missing enzymes.

Scientific Evidence

So far, there is no proof that dairy products cause arthritis. But there's some evidence they may contribute to rheumatoid arthritis and juvenile rheumatoid arthritis. Several studies and case histories show that when dairy is removed from the diet, inflammatory symptoms clear up for a few patients (Ratner, Panush 1, Parke).

Expert Opinion

If you want to check for a dairy sensitivity, it probably won't hurt most adults to eliminate dairy from their diet for a week or so, as long as they get adequate calcium from another source. However, some people with arthritis – such as post-menopausal women and anyone taking glucocorticoids – must be particularly careful about getting adequate calcium because of the increased risk of osteoporosis. Check with a doctor before you put a child or a teen on a dairy-free diet. These years are the peak times to build bone mass, and a calcium deficiency at these ages can increase osteoporosis risk in later years.

The Dong Diet

This restrictive diet was devised by Collin H. Dong, MD, to treat his own arthritis. It emphasizes all vegetables except tomatoes and eliminates many foods, including meat (except chicken), fruit, dairy, egg yolks, vinegar, pepper, chocolate, alcoholic and soft drinks, and all additives and preservatives. The diet was publicized in a book called *The Arthritic's Cookbook*.

Scientific Evidence

A study of people with arthritis that compared the Dong diet to a varied diet found no significant difference between the two. About half of those in each group felt better (Panush 2).

Expert Opinion

Some aspects – such as eliminating red meat – may help your overall health. However, this diet is of no proven benefit for arthritis or related musculoskeletal disorders. In fact, it may even be dangerous to your health if you try to follow the Dong diet for a long time.

Consulting a Dietitian

If you plan to consult a registered dietitian, look for one who has experience in or who specializes in your type of arthritis. Your rheumatologist may be able to refer you to a suitable dietitian, or you can get a list by calling the American Dietetic Association (see Resources). The usual fee is about $75 per hour, depending on where you live. It may be covered by insurance.

DIET CHANGES THAT MIGHT HELP

Vegetarian and Vegan Diets

More and more people these days are going vegetarian. Although many are vegetarians for ethical or environmental reasons, others – especially those with heart disease – are being advised by their physicians to cut down on animal products. Some choose a modified vegetarian diet that includes some animal products such as eggs (ovovegetarian), dairy products (lactovegetarian) and fish (pescovegetarian). A few choose a strict vegan diet that is completely plant-based, with no animal products of any kind.

Scientific Evidence

It's well-known that the high levels of saturated fat from meat can clog arteries and cause other heart disease. There's mixed evidence about whether eliminating saturated fat by following a vegetarian diet will help any form of arthritis.

In a randomized, controlled Scandinavian study, 27 adults with rheumatoid arthritis followed a vegan and gluten-free diet, while others ate an unrestricted diet. At the end of four weeks, the diet group had significantly improved, and a year later still had significant relief. A follow-up study of those who continued this diet showed the improvement continued two years later (Kjelsen-Hragh 1, Kjelsen-Hragh 2).

A randomized, controlled Finnish study of people with rheumatoid arthritis who ate a diet of uncooked vegan food with lactobacilli supplements (a type of "friendly" intestinal bacteria) showed a decrease in subjective symptoms for some (Nenonen). However, half of the people on the special diet experienced side effects including nausea and diarrhea and dropped out of the study.

Another type of vegetarian diet showed no positive results: A randomized, controlled study looked at the effects of fasting and a nine-week lactovegetarian diet on 16 people with rheumatoid arthritis. Although one-third showed reduced symptoms after fasting, only one person showed objective improvement on the lactovegetarian diet (Skoldstam 2).

Expert Opinion

A vegetarian diet may improve your overall health if not your arthritis. Vegetarian diets can increase your intake of antioxidants and vitamins because you'll be eating more fruits and vegetables. The lower fat level of the diet may help you lose weight, which can help ease pain from osteoarthritis of the knee. But remember that a completely vegan diet that cuts out *all* animal products may be inadequate in vitamins B6 and B12, which should be supplemented to prevent serious deficiency diseases.

Diet Advice for Gout, the Aristocratic Ache

So far, gout is the only form of arthritis that is proven to be linked to diet. For centuries, it was believed to be the curse of the royal and the well-to-do who indulged in rich foods, meats and alcoholic drinks.

Now scientists know that people with gout either have a defect in eliminating uric acid or make too much of it. Uric acid is a substance your body forms as a break-down product of purines. Purines come from foods such as meats and some fish. Purines are also made in your body. Normally, uric acid circulates in the bloodstream and is eliminated through the kidneys in the urine. In people with gout, uric acid builds up in the blood and forms sharp crystals that collect in your joints and soft tissues, causing inflammation and sometimes agonizing pain. The big toe is often the site of a gout attack. High levels of uric acid can also cause kidney stones. Although women do get gout after menopause, it is much more common in men.

Because gout can be controlled and seemingly often cured by drugs such as allopurinol and probenecid, most doctors have stopped recommending dietary changes. But you can help control gout by lowering the uric acid in your system through diet. Foods that have high levels of purines include meat and poultry (especially organ meats); dried beans and peas; anchovies, herring, mackerel, scallops and sardines; and asparagus, cauliflower, spinach and mushrooms. Avoiding or limiting these foods in your diet can contribute to the effectiveness of allopurinol or probenecid.

To help avoid gout attacks:

- Don't drink alcohol. Alcoholic beverages increase blood uric acid levels.
- Limit food with purines. These include meats and some seafoods (anchovies, herring, mackerel, scallops and sardines).
- Don't fast. Fasting increases the uric acid in your blood and can bring on an attack. If you are overweight, lose weight gradually.
- Drink water. Consume two to three quarts of water every day to help your body excrete uric acid.

Change Your Oil

An oil change in your diet may help you get better mileage out of your joints. Here are some recommendations from arthritis experts.

- You already get too much bad oil in fast food, restaurant foods and prepared foods. Get rid of the linoleic cooking and salad oils in your house such as corn, safflower and sunflower oils. Instead use olive oil, canola oil and flaxseed oil, which are high in beneficial fatty acids.

- Use more flaxseed in your diet. One to three tablespoons of oil a day is usual, and can be added to food. It can be used for salad dressings and some sautéing but not high-temperature cooking. You can also eat it as seed or meal. The Flaxseed Institute recommends about 30 grams of seed or meal a day. That's about a quarter of a cup per day. Flaxseed meal is like cornmeal in consistency and has a slightly nutty flavor. You can mix one or more tablespoons of the meal into breads; sprinkle it on cereal, salads or yogurt; stir it into soups; or add it to casseroles.

- Cut your meat, poultry and animal product consumption to no more than 4–6 ounces per day (about the size of a deck or two of playing cards). Wild game, free-grazing or range-raised meat that is not fattened with feed before slaughter is leaner and lower in omega-6 fatty acids.

- Add a cold water fish to your dinner menu two or three times a week. The fish can be fresh or frozen. Don't fry it – broil or bake it with no or little added fat.

- Remember that all fat – good or bad – has calories. Be sure to monitor your daily fat intake so that no more than 20–30 percent of your calories are from fat.

Certain vegetarian diets can be low in iron, vitamin B1 and calcium. To be nutritionally sound, a non-meat diet should be varied and supplemented with legumes (such as beans), nuts and a multivitamin with vitamin B12. Even a vegan diet can supply your nutritional needs, but takes more planning, and is not advised for young children. Consult your doctor and a dietitian for advice if you plan to go vegan, or consult a reputable book.

Balancing Fats in Your Diet

(See also Fish oil, Flaxseed, and Gamma linolenic acid, pages 209–212.)

We've all heard about the dangers of eating too much fat: It contributes to many diseases, and it also adds weight that can put more stress on your aching joints and muscles. Many of us are on low-fat diets recommended by our doctors. Therefore, it may come as a surprise to hear some doctors advocate *adding* oil in your diet to ease the symptoms of arthritis.

Actually, it's a question of balancing the types of fat in your diet. Researchers believe the kind of fat in the American diet is out of balance, and suggest you change the oils in your diet to improve your overall health as well as your arthritis symptoms. They recommend you eat more cold water fish and oils high in omega-3 fatty acids, and less of just about every other kind fat or oil. Here's why.

If you eat like a typical American, your diet is heavy with saturated fats from animal products that contribute to clogged arteries, cancer and many other ills. You are also probably eating too much of the omega-6 linoleic fatty acids that contribute to inflammation, and too little of the omega-3 fatty acids.

The omega fatty acids are essential for survival, and we have to get them from foods. But most of us have diets overwhelmed with the omego-6 fatty acids that form linoleic acid and fuel inflammation. Linoleic acids are found in most vegetable oils such as corn and safflower, are used in processed and fast foods, and are in our corn-fattened meat supply as well. These are converted into arachidonic acids that provide the building blocks for the leukotrienes and series 2 prostaglandins that cause inflammation and pain in arthritis.

The omega-3 fatty acids, on the other hand, fight inflammation. They contain eicosapentaenoic acid (EPA) and docosahexaenoic acid (DHA), fatty acids that compete with arachidonic acids. EPA and DHA supply the chemical building blocks to make the series 1 and 3 prostaglandins and leukotrienes that reduce inflammation. They also help keep your blood thinner and improve circulation (see Fish oil, page 209).

Humans used to get a lot more of the omega-3 type fatty acids because we ate wild greens, whole grains, seeds and the wild game that fed on these. Today, most Americans don't get enough omega-3 oils in their diet to balance out that flood of linoleic fatty acids.

Changing the balance of fats in your diet may help your rheumatoid arthritis symptoms – and also improve your heart health and help prevent cancer. The best source of omega-3 is in cold water fish (see page 172). Another good source of EPA is flaxseed, which can be found as a cooking oil and as a meal used in baking (see Flaxseed, page 211). Flaxseed breaks down into EPA, and it also contains lignans, which may help prevent breast and colon cancer. Canola and olive oils also have a better balance of fatty acids.

There is another fatty acid that has had good results fighting inflammation, but it

Foods that Give Good Fat

Here are some foods with relatively high levels of omega-3 fatty acids. In general, the colder the water, the more omega-3 oil in the fish. Be sure they are wild: Farm-raised fish (such as some salmon) are fed commercial products that lower the omega-3 levels.

Food	Grams of omega-3 per 3.5-ounce serving
Sardines* (in their own oil)	21.1
Butternuts (white walnuts)* (dried)	8.7
Black walnuts*	3.3
Green soybeans	3.2
Mackerel*	2.5
Herring*	1.7
Trout (lake)	1.6
Anchovy	1.4
Sablefish*	1.4
Salmon	1.2
Bluefish	1.2
Mullet	1.1

Information provided by the Nutrition Department, Pennsylvania State University.
* These items are high in total fat content.

doesn't occur in large amounts in most foods. It's called gamma-linolenic acid (GLA), and it's found concentrated in borage oil, evening primrose oil and black currant seed oil (See Gamma-linolenic acids, page 212). GLA helps produce series 1 prostaglandins that fight inflammation.

Scientific Evidence

The research is promising. More than a dozen studies show concentrated fish oil supplements can ease the aches of rheumatoid arthritis, and one study showed it helped Raynaud's phenomenon (Kremer, DiCiacomo). Other studies have shown that evening primrose oil and borage oil relieve rheumatoid arthritis also, perhaps even better than fish oil (Belch, Leventhal).

Expert Opinion

Omega-3 and GLA oil supplements have been shown to reduce inflammation. To get enough of these healing oils, however, you have to swallow a lot of capsules. And although they aren't expensive compared to many drugs, they aren't cheap either, and they are not likely to be covered by insurance.

However, you can combine some oil supplements with diet changes, and improve your overall health by changing the balance of the oils in your diet. Eat fewer animal products and use less linoleic-rich oils – and eat more fish and consider adding flaxseed products.

Cautions

! Do not try diet changes if you are pregnant or nursing, or likely to become pregnant.

! Do not experiment with restrictive diets for children, the elderly or those with severe arthritis. Food deficiencies in childhood can cause permanent damage to growing children, especially babies. Older people, those who are seriously ill and people on multiple medications are also more at risk of dietary deficiencies. Ask your health professional to recommend a registered dietitian.

Good Advice

Some common sense approaches can help your whole health, not just your arthritis.

- Before you start eliminating foods, look at your overall diet and see if you can make some healthy choices for yourself and your family. Start by cutting out – or cutting down on – junk food, fast food, high-fat foods, alcohol, sodas, coffee, tea, sugar and sugar-rich deserts and, of course, tobacco use.

- Get into the five-a-day program. Eat five servings a day of fruits or vegetables. It's easy to do, for your whole family. Have a banana with cereal or a grapefruit half for breakfast, a fruit snack at midday. An 8-ounce glass of juice is one serving, so drink juice instead of soda. (Be sure to read the labels: Not all prepared juices are 100 percent juice.)

- Eat more broccoli and other dark green vegetables called crucifers, especially if you have lupus. Some experts believe these help balance hormones.

- Explore soy. It is a prime source of protein. Green soybeans are high in omega-3 fatty acids, and some animal studies show soy appears to ease pain. Tofu is the ultimate boring food, it's true: It has no color, no texture and no taste, which is great. You can make it taste like anything.

- Plan your poisons. You want to indulge in a food that causes problems. You know you'll pay. Do it with awareness, and you'll probably do it less often.

- Keep a food diary for a month of what you eat and how you feel, and see if you notice a difference with certain foods.

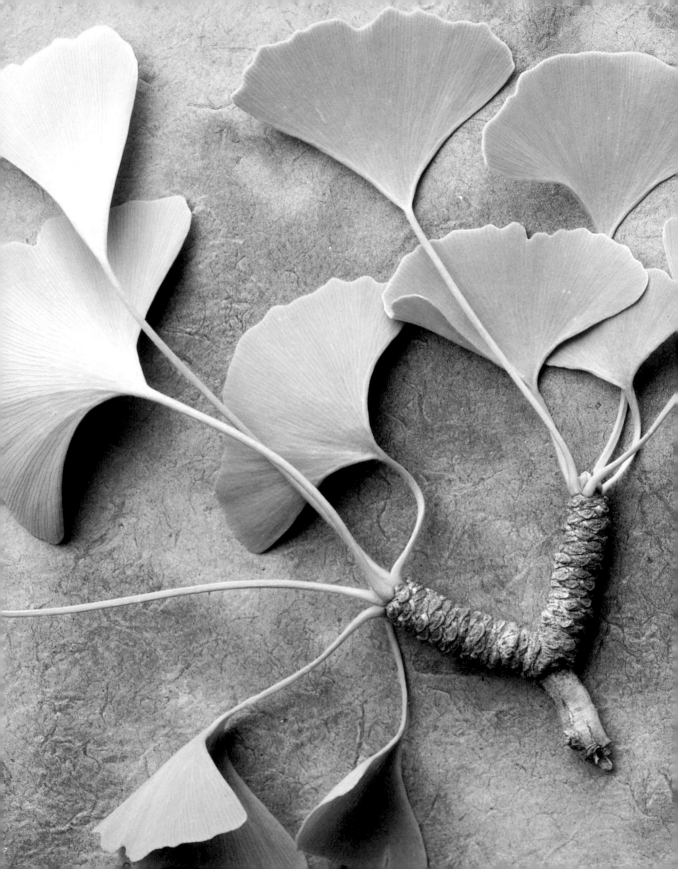

Nature's Remedies

HERBS AND SUPPLEMENTS FOR ARTHRITIS

Look in the medicine cabinet of just about anybody with arthritis these days, and the supplements will be crowding out the prescription drugs. And we're not talking about multivitamins: These supplements include herbs, minerals, enzymes and an array of more exotic remedies – and some of them are there with a doctor's blessing.

That's a big change from a few decades ago when herbs and supplements were something used by health nuts and hippies, and considered about as useful as snake oil. Today's supplement users tend to be well-educated, middle-class, middle-aged – and willing to pay out-of-pocket for unproven remedies. In 1997, they spent nearly $12 billion on herbal and dietary supplement products, according to market researchers.

Herbs and supplements have a tremendous appeal for people with arthritis and related diseases who are frustrated with the inability of conventional medicine to cure their disease or fully relieve their symptoms. And many of the conventional medications have side effects that require yet more medication to counter or control. Supplements offer the convenience of popping a pill or potion along with the premise that the "natural" ingredients will heal without harming – or at least with fewer side effects than the potent prescription drugs so many are taking for arthritis.

But natural doesn't always mean safe. Some people think that supplements – especially herbs – are safe because they are "natural" alternatives to the chemicals in prescription drugs. Fact is, herbs are chemicals. And anything that's strong enough to help is also strong enough to hurt.

There's not a lot of solid scientific information about herbs and supplements, and they are not regulated as medical products to make sure they are effective – or even safe. When you use them, you're forging off into uncharted territory. And your usual sources of information probably can't help. Most doctors and pharmacists are suspicious of herbs and supplements because there are no purity standards or quality control mechanisms. And, they admit, they don't know much about them. So if you want to prescribe for yourself, you're going to have to do your own research. And that presents another problem: Even though millions of people are taking supplements every day, there just isn't much solid scientific evidence about what most of them do.

A few supplements, such as vitamin C and St. John's wort, have been well studied. But for most there are few studies, and many of the ones that do exist don't stand up to rigorous scientific examination.

The Good News about Natural Products

Natural products were our first medicines, and are the source of at least 25 percent of today's drugs, with more being discovered. Aspirin came from willow bark, penicillin from mold, digitalis from a garden plant called foxglove. The cancer drug taxol is from yew bark, opium comes from Oriental poppies, and a promising new pain drug being developed was discovered in the venom of a South American frog. In much of the world, botanical and other products from nature still are the medicine, not the alternative.

Overall, herbs are more complex and have milder effects than prescription drugs. Supplements often contain the entire plant, which has many active ingredients. In drugs, the active ingredient has usually been isolated and concentrated to give a more powerful effect. Our potent modern drugs get fast results, which is good for an acute or life-threatening illness. But they also often have pretty potent side effects, which is a concern for those with chronic ailments who will be taking them for years.

Although we need more evidence, studies are suggesting that some supplements may ease some arthritis symptoms.

Proceeding with Caution

Health food and nutrition stores, pharmacies – even supermarkets – are crowded with slick-looking supplements packaged in just about every form you can imagine, from tinctures and teas to tablets, capsules, ointments, sprays and even skin patches. People who were wary of raw herbs and folk medicine are now buying shrink-wrapped prepackaged pills, potions and capsules that have the same ingredients but look as safe as regulated over-the-counter drugs.

The truth is, these preparations are no more regulated than raw herbs. Because supplements are so professionally packaged, you may not know that these products haven't been tested for safety or effectiveness. Under the Dietary Supplement Health and Education Act (DSHEA) of 1994, products sold as "dietary supplements" don't have to pass any tests to prove they are effective – or even safe. They can only be removed from the market after it's shown they are harmful. That's a major difference from Food and Drug Administration (FDA)-approved prescription and over-the-counter drugs, which have to be proven safe or effective before they go on the market. (Two exceptions: Homeopathic remedies and vitamins are FDA-approved.)

Reading the Labels

Some manufacturers of dietary supplements have been giving good label information to consumers for years. Now the law requires it on all dietary supplements. Starting in 1999, manufacturers must put **"Supplement Facts"** information on their labels, similar to the "Nutritional Facts" panels you see on foods. They must now specify the active ingredients, with other ingredients in descending order of predominance, and list them by common name along with the serving size.

Supplement Facts		
Serving Size 1 Capsule		
Amount Per Capsules		**% Daily Value**
Calories 20		
Calories from Fat 20		
Total Fat 2 g		
Saturated Fat 0.5 g		3%*
Polyunsaturated Fat 1 g		3%*
Monounsaturated Fat 0.5 g		†
Vitamin A 4250 IU		†
Vitamin D 425 IU		65%
		100%
Omega-3 fatty acids 0.5 g		†

* Percent Daily Values are based on a 2,000 calorie diet.
† Daily Value not established.

Ingredients: Cod liver oil, gelatin, water, and glycerin.

Other information required on the labels of dietary supplements includes the total quantity of contents (such as "60 capsules"); directions for use; the name and place of business of manufacturer, packer or distributor (this is the address to write for more product information). Along with any claim for function or effect, the label also has to say "This statement has not been evaluated by the Food and Drug Administration. This product is not intended to diagnose, treat, cure, or prevent any disease."

You can see what a proper label should look like on the FDA Web site at www.fda.gov.

The DSHEA law is credited with the explosive growth of the supplement industry. About the only regulation on dietary supplements is that vendors can't claim their products treat, cure, diagnose or prevent disease. That's why you'll see carefully worded labels full of double-talk. An OA supplement, for example, can't legally claim to "replace damaged cartilage from osteoarthritis" but can claim to "support healthy joints." (See Reading the Labels.)

This lack of regulation also means there's no guarantee the bottle you buy has what the label says, or as much as it says, or is free of toxins or additives. That's especially true of herbal products: They come from plants, and every gardener knows the quality of plant products depends on how, where and when they were grown, harvested, stored and packaged. The active ingredients can vary greatly, and – although it happens rarely – anywhere along the line they can become polluted with heavy metals, chemicals or bacteria. People have died from reactions to herbs. In November 1998, the *New England Journal of Medicine* reported on bad incidents with herbs that included lead poisoning.

The sales staff selling these products generally know little more than you do. In some cases, they know a lot less, but that doesn't stop them from enthusiastically offering advice. When *Arthritis Today* editors went shopping for dietary supplements, they found salesclerks eager to "prescribe" for arthritis. But only one of 14 salesclerks asked what kind of arthritis. All the rest were unaware that arthritis is an umbrella term for more than 100 diseases, and offered treatments for the only one they knew of: osteoarthritis.

If this is making you more cautious about using supplements, it should. Supplements have great potential, but there's just not much consumer protection. You are really on your own here until scientific studies are completed that add to our knowledge about the effects of herbs and supplements on arthritis.

The hard facts are that when you take a product that hasn't been tested and proven safe and effective, you're conducting your own scientific experiment – and you're the guinea pig. If you are going to be your own doctor, observe the basic principle of the Hippocratic oath: First do no harm.

This chapter reviews the supplements most-used or recommended for rheumatic diseases, and gives the available scientific evidence, an expert opinion, cautions and information on how the supplement is used. There's a section about herb-drug interactions as well – but not all of them will be listed, because all of them aren't known. For the same reason, if you don't see an item here, it's because we didn't find enough information to be able to offer an opinion.

Finding the Safest Supplements

The explosion of interest in herbs and dietary supplements can be seen in the huge number of suppliers that have entered the marketplace. Some are very good, and others aren't. How do you tell the difference and get good quality products?

- Begin by asking your doctor or other health professionals what they recommend. Ask if they can help you find out which brands are most dependable.
- Buy from large national companies,

pharmacies or health food stores that have a major investment in maintaining their reputations. They are likely to be concerned about quality and safety.

- Look for products with the U.S.P. notation, which indicates the manufacturer followed standards established by the United States Pharmacopoeia.
- Use European brands, or their United States versions. Doctors advise buying herbs that originate in Europe, especially Germany where herbal remedies are carefully regulated.
- Don't buy through the mail or over the Internet unless you know the vendor is reputable and will stand by its products.
- Avoid products that are backed only with testimonials. You want scientific research, not opinion. Beware of any product that promises to do too much. If it sounds too good to be true, it probably is.
- When a company advertises that a supplement has been "scientifically studied" or "scientifically proven," contact them and ask to receive copies of the studies. If they can't or won't send them, don't buy this brand.
- When a supplement has been studied with good results,

find out which brand was used in the study, and buy that. It may take some work to find out this information. Ask your local reference librarian for help (see Looking at the Scientific Evidence, page 14).

Finding a Practitioner for Herbs and Supplements

It's difficult to find qualified herbal practitioners. Currently, there is no state or federal certification process or licensing for the practice of herbal medicine. In some states, licensed naturopathic physicians and some licensed acupuncturists can dispense herbs for medicinal use. Generally, it is illegal for anyone who is not a licensed health professional to practice medicine with herbs.

Few pharmacists or doctors know much about dietary supplements or herbs. An article in *The Archives of Internal Medicine* reports that the American medical establishment has a bias against vitamins in spite of evidence that shows vitamin and mineral supplements can help with many conditions.

One way to change this is to urge your doctors and pharmacists to learn more about herbs and supplements so they can better advise you and other patients about the products flooding the marketplace. Show them the citations from medical journals that go with this chapter, and encourage them to form a relationship with those who have expertise in supplement use.

Understanding the Terms

Going off to buy a supplement is an ordeal. You're likely to find it in a dozen different brands, formulations and forms. It may come as a tea, tincture, capsule, liquid or spray. And if you go on the Internet, the possibilities can overwhelm you.

Some companies promise **standardized products**, meaning that each dose in a batch has the same ingredients in the same amounts. Look for this on the label. It's your best assurance that the product has what it claims, and it gives the percentage of the key (or active) ingredients. But it's no guarantee, because nutritional supplements aren't regulated. The quality applies only to that one batch, not all the products of that kind made by that company. Some organizations and the FDA are working toward establishing good manufacturing practices.

Raw herbs are fresh or dried plant parts that the user prepares at home in various ways. While this seems the most natural way, often these botanicals have lost their medical potency because they've gotten old and have been exposed to air. Of course, if they are fresh-picked they will still be potent. You may also find freeze-dried herbs, which are fresher than air-dried.

More often, herbs are sold as **extracts**, which are concentrated forms of herbs or plants prepared in capsules or tablets. **Tinctures** are liquid extracts of herbs, usually in alcohol. You dilute them before use by adding the specified amount to water. **Infusions** are teas or liquids made by soaking or cooking botanicals in water. By the way, most supermarket herbal teas – those prettily packaged tea bags you find on the grocery shelves – don't have enough strength to help or hurt you. They're mainly beverage teas with no medicinal value.

Supplements come in capsules or tablets, and you face similar problems in finding a pure, safe product. When you want to be sure you're getting a pure product, such as DHEA or DMSO, ask your doctor to give you a prescription to a **compounding pharmacy**. These are specialty pharmacies that make up custom medicinals. They can also make up products without any additives. It will cost more – sometimes a bit more, sometimes a lot – but you know what you're getting (see Resources).

Meanwhile, here are your best bets in finding a practitioner.

Osteopathic and Naturopathic Physicians

Many naturopathic doctors (NDs), but not all, have extensive experience with herbs and supplements. Some osteopathic physicians also use complementary therapies. Ask about expertise, or for a referral to an expert (see Osteopathic Medicine, page 40; and Naturopathic Medicine, page 37).

Practitioners of Chinese and Ayurvedic Medicine

Some Chinese medicine practitioners are certified in Asian herbal use but licensed in only a few states to prescribe herbs (see Chinese Medicine, page 33). Similarly, ayurvedic physicians use Indian herbs (see Ayurveda, page 29). However, there are few qualified practitioners in the United States.

Medical Doctors

Some physicians with an interest in complementary medicine may be informed. It's not likely that an MD will also be an herbalist, but an increasing number of doctors are interested in using herbs and supplements in their practice, and are willing to work with an herbalist. Look for doctors who say they practice holistic or integrative medicine (see How to Find a Complementary Medical Practitioner, page 18).

Pharmacists

Although pharmacists learn something about herbs and supplements while in school, they generally aren't well-educated about the use of most dietary supplements. They may be able to help you: Ask. Some chain pharmacy companies that carry a wide range of supplements are training their pharmacists.

Herbalists

You take potluck here, because anyone can claim to be an expert. Many herbalists learn through apprenticeship with an expert, which can take many years. Some are graduates of excellent European herbal training programs, so ask about training and certification, if any. Look for an herbalist who works with an MD, naturopath or other health professional.

Other Health Professionals

Chiropractors and many other health professionals will prescribe herbs and supplements for you. Their expertise varies widely. Ask about their training and certification in supplement use.

Cautions

! Always tell your doctor everything you're taking. Although most won't offer usage recommendations, they may know about potential interactions with the drugs you

Although some of the substances described here have been used for hundreds or even thousands of years in traditional medicines, few have been adequately studied with modern scientific methods. There is little evidence to show what they are actually doing to your body. Should you decide to take these unregulated substances, be aware that you are experimenting. Be sure to tell your doctor, and be alert to any side effects or problems.

If you don't find a substance listed here, it's because we didn't find enough evidence for or against it to be able to offer any information.

are already taking, as well as any particular dangers or reports of ill effects.

! If you are pregnant or breastfeeding, don't take anything without asking your doctor first: Some supplements can cause birth defects or harm your baby.

! Don't give supplements to children or the elderly without professional advice.

! If you have any side effects, stop taking the supplement right away and call your doctor.

! Don't take any supplement for more than three months without a medical evaluation. Remember: What's OK for someone in good health may not be a good idea for someone with an illness, especially those taking other medications. See your physician for an examination to check for side effects – and to see if there is any improvement that makes it worth continuing using it.

! Don't take massive doses. More is not better – and you can overdose on anything, no matter how "safe" it appears to be.

! Be aware of drug interactions: Ask your doctor or pharmacist about possible interactions with the prescription drugs you are taking (see Potential Supplement-Drug Interactions, page 235).

Good Advice

• Spending a bundle on supplements and herbs can't make up for stress, lack of exercise, poor sleep habits, a lousy diet, and use of addictive and damaging substances such as tobacco, alcohol, caffeine and recreational drugs. Before you head to the health food store, consider investing instead in lifestyle changes that can improve your health and well-being without any side effects.

• Get a diagnosis from a doctor before you start self-medicating. One of the dangers of

Organizations

American Botanical Council
P.O. Box 144345
Austin, TX 78714-4345
Phone: 512/926-4900
E-mail: abc@herbalgram.org
Web site: http://www.herbalgram.org
A nonprofit research and education organization that focuses on the uses of herbs and plant-based medicines. Publishes the peer-reviewed journal *HerbalGram* in coordination with the Herb Research Foundation (see below), and many other educational books and materials on herbs.

American Dietetic Association
216 West Jackson Boulevard
Chicago, IL 60606-6995
Phone: 800/366-1655 for recorded messages and referrals to a registered dietitian, or 900/225-5267 to talk to a registered dietitian. There's a charge of $1.95 for the first minute, $0.95 for each additional minute.
Web site: http://www.eatright.org

American Herbalists Guild
P.O. Box 70, Roosevelt, UT 84066.
Phone: 435/722-8434
E-mail: ahgoffice@earthlink.net
Web site: http://www.healthy.net/herbalists
Has referrals to herbal practitioners.

Council for Responsible Nutrition
1875 I Street, NW, Suite 400
Washington, DC 20006-5409
Phone: 202/872-1488
Web site: http://www.crnusa.org
This trade association represents nutritional supplement companies. It provides consumer information by phone, mail or online at its Web site.

The Herb Research Foundation
1007 Pearl Street, Suite 200
Boulder, CO 80302
Phone: 800/748-2617 or 303/449-2265
E-mail: info@herbs.org
Web site: http://www.herbs.org/index.html
HRF is a nonprofit research and educational organization focusing on herbs and medicinal plants.

International Academy of Compounding Pharmacists
Phone: 800/927-4227
Compounding pharmacies make a prescription from scratch to your doctor's order, using U.S.P. grade pure chemicals. Most prescriptions will cost more, but you'll be guaranteed a safe source for supplements such as DHEA. Your doctor can also order drugs made without additives, such as corn or sugar. The IACP has 1,200 members, and can refer you or your doctor to a member in your area.

Federal Agencies

Food and Drug Administration
Office of Consumer Affairs, HFE-88
Rockville, MD 20857
Food Information Phone Line:
800/FDA-4010
To ask about a product: 888/463-6332
Web site: http://www.fda.gov/opacom/morecons.html

FDA Adverse Event Monitoring System
http://www.cfsan.fda.gov/~dms/aems.html
Reports associated with use of a nutritional product such as dietary supplements (includes herbs), infant formulas and medical foods.

FDA Center for Food Safety and Applied Nutrition
E-mail: execsec@oc.fda.gov
Web site: http://vm.cfsan.fda.gov
Regulates foods and dietary supplements; issues warnings of dangerous products.

"An FDA Guide to Dietary Supplements"
An online article at:
http://vm.cfsan.fda.gov/~dms/fdsupp.html

IBIDS (International Bibliographic Information on Dietary Supplements)
An online database of published scientific literature on dietary supplements, including vitamins, minerals and botanicals.
Web site: http://odp.od.nih.gov/ods/databases/ibids.html

National Center for Complementary and Alternative Medicine Clearinghouse
P.O. Box 8218
Silver Spring, MD 20907-8218
Phone: 888/644-6226
Web site: http://nccam.nih.gov
This source is mainly focused on NCCAM-funded research, but will help you find other sources for alternative therapies and remedies.

NIH Office of Dietary Supplements
Web site: http://dietary-supplements.info.nih.gov

USDA Food and Nutrition Information Center
Agricultural Research Service, USDA
National Agricultural Library, Room 301
10301 Baltimore Avenue
Beltsville, MD 20705-2351
Phone: 301/504-5719
Web site: http://www.nal.usda.gov/fnic

treating yourself with supplements is that you might miss signs of serious illness that requires conventional medical treatment. Before you go shopping for a cure, be sure you know what you are trying to treat.

- Be careful whose advice you take. Don't depend on sales staff for medical advice. While eager to "prescribe," the salespeople in health food stores know little about the full effects of their products. Find an expert to help you choose types of supplements and doses. This can be difficult but your doctor or pharmacist may be able to help you. (see Finding a Practitioner)

- If you are self-prescribing, try products one at a time so you can assess the effect — or lack of any. Keep daily notes of how it seems to be effecting you.

- Look for warnings on the supplement label or in a good reference book, especially for interactions with other over-the-counter or prescription drugs you may be taking.

Books

Be wary of books on herbs and supplements that give lots of information, but don't cite any medical references or sources.

Encyclopedia of Natural Medicine, Revised 2nd Edition, by Michael Murray, ND, and Joseph Pizzorno, ND. 1998. Rocklin, CA. Prima Publishing. Paperback. $24.95.
Good information in the tradition of naturopathic medicine, with medical journal references and other excellent sources.

The Essential Guide for Improving Your Health Naturally, by Michael T. Murray. 1996. Rocklin, CA. Prima Publishing. Paperback. $19.95.
Solid information on supplements with medical journal references, but doesn't include herbs or a section on fibromyalgia.

Herbal Medicine: The Expanded Commission E Monographs, edited by Mark Blumenthal and Alicia Goldberg. 1999. Boston: Integrative Medicine Communications. $59.
Evaluations on the safety and efficacy of botanicals by the expert panel appointed by Germany's equivalent of the Food and Drug Administration. This scholarly tome is heavy reading, but a useful reference.

Herbs of Choice: The Therapeutic Use of Phytomedicinals, by Varro E. Tyler, PhD. 1994. The Haworth Press, Inc. Paperback. $24.95.

The Green Pharmacy, by James A. Duke, PhD. 1998. New York. Tor Books. Paperback. $6.99.
A survey of herbs based mostly on folk traditions and botany with pithy comments by this retired USDA herbalist and syndicated columnist. Doesn't cite medical journal sources.

The Natural Pharmacy: From the Top Experts in the Field, Your Essential Guide to Vitamins, Herbs, Minerals and Homeopathic Remedies, by Skye Lininger, DC, et al. 1998. Rocklin, CA. Prima Health. Paperback. $19.95. Also available on CD-ROM.
A review of herbs and supplements with medical journal references.

The Professional's Handbook of Complementary & Alternative Therapies, by Charles W. Fetrow and Juan R. Avila. 1999. Springhouse. $36.95.
Compiled by two doctors of pharmacy, this gives solid information from medical studies on herbs and supplements.

Tyler's Honest Herbal: A Sensible Guide to the Use of Herbs and Related Remedies, by Varro E. Tyler, PhD, and Steven Foster. 1998. The Haworth Press, Inc. Hardcover. $49.95.

What the Labels Won't Tell You: A Consumer Guide to Herbal Supplements, by Logan V. Chamberlain. 1998. Interweave Press. Paperback. $9.95.

Web Sites

These Web sites offer information about botanicals and dietary supplements. Be aware that online addresses and contents change frequently. Listing these sites does not imply approval of the content by the Arthritis Foundation.

American Botanical Council
Web site: http://www.herbalgram.org

American Herbal Products Association
Web site: http://www.ahpa.org

Council for Responsible Nutrition
Web site: http://www.crnusa.org

Dr. Duke's Phytochemical and Ethnobotanical Databases
Web site: http://www.ars-grin.gov/duke
Botanist James Duke's home page and entry into a database of the chemical composition and uses of many botanicals. It is not for the dabbler.

HerbMed
Web site: http://www.amfoundation.org/_vti_bin/shtml.exe/herbmed.htm
An excellent electronic herbal database that provides hyperlinked access to scientific data on herbs for health for professionals, researchers and the general public. The number of herbs included is small, but growing. HerbMed is a project of the Alternative Medicine Foundation, Inc.

Herb Research Foundation
Web site: http://www.herbs.org/contact.html

Institute for Nutraceutical Advancement
Web site: http://www.nutraceuticalinstitute.com

The Institute for Traditional Medicine
Web site: http://itmonline.org
A nonprofit educational institution offering programs with a focus on natural healing.

MedHerb.com from Medical Herbalism
Web site: http://www.medherb.com
A medical herbalism site with many links and databases.

Medical Herbalism Online Materia Medica
Web site: http://www.medherb.com/MATMED.HTM
Describes many herbs and traditional uses, with illustrations.

Mother Nature.com
Web site: http://www.mothernature.com
This is a commercial site that sells alternative health products. It contains an excellent "Encyclopedia of Natural Health" that includes a guide to herbs and supplements that cites medical studies; and a list of drug-herb-vitamin-supplement interactions.

Organic Trade Association
Web site: http://www.ota.com/top.htm

Herbs and Supplements and Their Uses
Read individual entries to learn about the research behind the claims.

THERAPY	PAIN	STIFFNESS	FATIGUE	INFLAMMATION	ANXIETY/DEPRESSION	USES AND COMMENTS
ALOE	●			●		Topical use; not advised for internal use
ASU	●	●				For OA
AYURVEDIC REMEDIES	●	●	●	●		Herbs used in combinations for many conditions
BLACK CURRANT OIL	●	●		●		For RA; see GLA
BORAGE OIL	●	●		●		For RA; see GLA
BORON	●	●		●		For RA, OA; may raise estrogen levels
BOSWELLIA	●	●		●		For RA, OA; often used in combinations
BROMELAIN				●		Not enough evidence
CAT'S CLAW	●			●		For RA; animal studies only; may protect GI tract
CAYENNE	●					Topical use; recommended
CHINESE HERBS	●	●	●	●		Herbs used in combinations for many conditions
CHONDROITIN SULFATE	●	●				For OA
CMO						No human studies; not recommended
COLLAGEN	●	●		●		For RA; not the same as cartilage
COPPER	●			●		Not enough evidence
CURCUMIN	●	●		●		For RA, OA; often used in combinations
DEVIL'S CLAW						No evidence it helps RA
DHEA	●		●	●		For lupus; don't use without physician's help
DMSO	●	●		●		Don't use without physician's help
ECHINACEA						Not recommended for autoimmune disease
ELEUTHERO			●			See ginseng
EVENING PRIMROSE OIL	●	●		●		For RA; see GLA
FISH OIL	●	●	●	●	●	For RA, Raynaud's

THERAPY	PAIN	STIFFNESS	FATIGUE	INFLAMMATION	ANXIETY/DEPRESSION	USES AND COMMENTS
FLAXSEED	●	●		●		For RA, possibly lupus nephritis, constipation
GIN-SOAKED RAISINS						Not recommended
GINGER	●			●		For RA, OA; relieves nausea
GINKO						May improve circulation in Raynaud's
GINSENG			●			
GLA	●	●		●		For RA
GLUCOSAMINE	●	●				For OA
GREEN TEA	●			●		Cancer protector; no human studies for arthritis
GUAIFENESIN						Touted for fibromyalgia; not recommended
KAVA KAVA	●				●	Relaxant; don't use with alcohol or depression drugs
MAGNESIUM	●			●		For fibromyalgia and chronic fatigue
MELATONIN						Enhances sleep; not recommended for autoimmune diseases
MSM	●			●		No human studies
SAM	●	●			●	For OA, depression, fibromyalgia
ST. JOHN'S WORT					●	Not for serious depression
SELENIUM	●	●		●		For RA
STINGING NETTLE	●	●		●		For RA, OA; enhances NSAID effectiveness
THUNDER GOD VINE	●			●		For RA, autoimmune diseases; not enough evidence
TURMERIC	●	●		●		For RA, OA; often used in combinations
VALERIAN						Enhances sleep; don't use with alcohol or depression drugs
VITAMINS						See page 231
WILD YAM						Not recomended
ZINC SULFATE	●	●		●		For RA, psoriasis

ALOE *(Aloe vera, Aloe barbadensis)*

The aloe plant has been used medicinally for thousands of years to treat wounds and for gastrointestinal problems. Most of us are familiar with its external use. The flesh of aloe leaves, used fresh or prepared in a gel, soothes burns and scrapes and is known to reduce inflammation and promote healing (Heggers). In fact, an aloe plant is a common fixture in many kitchens as first aid for minor burns.

Aloe is also marketed for internal use to treat rheumatoid arthritis, and as a laxative. Two different parts of the leaf are used for these very different purposes. The aloe gel from the center of the leaf (sometimes called juice) is made into drinks recommended for everything from ulcers to arthritis, and marketed as an energizing tonic. Aloe material taken from just inside the skin contains anthraquinones, a powerful purgative. This is an FDA-approved laxative.

There is animal evidence for internal use of aloe gel for inflammation. Rats injected with fresh, whole *Aloe vera* leaf were protected from developing an artificially induced rheumatoid arthritis, or had less inflammation (Hanley). In another study, mice with wounds who got aloe both in drinking water and applied to the sore area healed more quickly (Davis).

However, there is no acceptable scientific evidence in humans to show that aloe gel taken internally will relieve arthritis – and it may have risks. If the leaf products aren't carefully separated, the aloe gel may contain the purgative anthraquinones, which can have powerful effects and can cause intestinal pain and damage. There's also no guarantee that processed aloe gel products will have the active ingredients of fresh aloe gel.

How It's Used

Aloe is sold for internal and external use. When used externally, aloe gel – or sometimes a whole fresh leaf – is placed on burns or other wounds. It is available in shampoos and other hair products, lip moisturizers, soaps, sunscreens, and facial tissues. Aloe is also sold in lotions for arthritis pain, sometimes combined with other ingredients.

When used internally, aloe is marketed for two very different uses. Dried aloe concentrate from the lining of the leaf is sold in capsules as a laxative. The usual dosage is 50-200 mg per day. Aloe gel is available in varying concentrations in drinks. The dosage varies.

Expert Opinion

There's good documentation that aloe applied externally can speed the healing of shallow wounds and burns and help many skin conditions (including sunburn and psoriasis). But most experts don't recommend aloe gel for internal use. There's just not enough scientific evidence to show it's safe – or that it's effective enough to be worth taking a risk.

Cautions

! Do not use aloe gel on deep wounds, because it may slow healing.

! Do not have aloe injections.

! Be aware that aloe laxatives are powerful: They can cause severe abdominal pain and overdoses can cause bleeding and diarrhea.

! Taken during pregnancy, aloe may cause uterine contractions and miscarriage.

! Some sources say aloe taken internally may increase the effects of several drugs, including glucocorticoids.

Good Advice

• Check labels of aloe gel or juice sold for internal use: It should be pasteurized and prepared with preservatives to prevent contamination.

AVOCADO/SOYBEAN OIL

A mixture of oils from avocado and soybeans called ASU (avocado/soybean unsaponifiables) shows promise for relieving osteoarthritis pain.

In 1998, a team of French scientists studied 164 people with severe osteoarthritis of the knee or hip in a double-blind, placebo-controlled trial. For six months, 85 took capsules with 300 mg of ASU and the rest took a placebo. Although both groups improved, the ASU group showed significantly less pain and disability than those taking placebo (Maheu). A similar study found that those taking ASU for three months needed fewer NSAIDs to control pain than the placebo group (Blotman). A test tube study suggests ASU might prompt cartilage growth (Boumediene).

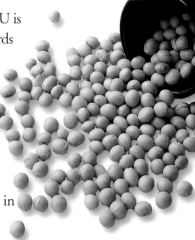

The ratio of the oils in ASU is one-third avocado to two-thirds soybean, and the action appears to depend on the mixture. It is believed to help stimulate cartilage repair, but the exact way it works isn't understood yet.

The product is marketed in

France (where the studies were done) and several other countries as *Plascledine 300*. It was not available in the United States at the time of publication, but could be sold here soon.

How It's Used

The compound was given in 300-mg capsules once a day.

Expert Opinion

This combination is worth a try. Studies have shown a consistent positive effect for osteoarthritis.

Cautions

! There were no serious side effects from the treatment.

AYURVEDIC REMEDIES

See Ginger, Turmeric, Boswellia

The ancient Indian healing system of ayurveda uses herbs, minerals and other remedies to enhance health as well as heal illness (see Ayurveda, page 27). Many of these herbs won't be familiar to you. They aren't found outside of Asia, and their names may be in Sanskrit. Others, such as ginger, are well-known.

Remedies are almost always given in combinations, prescribed – and often prepared – specifically for you and your individual situation. These remedies are also available in standardized formulations for arthritis. There are too many combinations to discuss here, and many have not been studied outside Asia. Evidence shows that some of these remedies relieve inflammation and ease the pains of arthritis. Among these are ginger, boswellia, turmeric and ashwaghanda. In randomized controlled trials, a combination of these four herbs showed promise for relieving symptoms of both osteoarthritis and rheumatoid arthritis (Chopra 1, Chopra 2).

Other traditional remedies may include minerals or heavy metals such as lead or mercury that are specially treated. However, these are not often used today and you are not likely to encounter them in the United States.

Expert Opinion

Ayurvedic remedies have been used for thousands of years, and are often given along with instructions for lifestyle and dietary changes that can improve your health. Look for a practitioner experienced in ayurvedic remedies if you decide to try them and ask about possible interactions and side effects.

Cautions

! Ayurvedic herbs and remedies should be used with caution because they are not regulated as medications, and because some traditional remedies may contain heavy metals.

! Some remedies intensify the effects of drugs or other herbs. Check with your physician before starting.

BLACK CURRANT OIL

See GLA (gamma linolenic acids)

BORAGE OIL

See GLA (gamma linolenic acids)

BORON

Boron is a trace mineral that helps us use calcium and magnesium, and that could be important to bone and joint health. It also has anti-inflammatory actions, and there is some evidence boron supplements can case symptoms for those with osteoporosis, osteoarthritis and rheumatoid arthritis (Newnham).

In an animal study, boron supplements significantly reduced rheumatoid arthritis-like effects in rats and doubled their natural killer cell concentrations (Hunt). Humans given boron saw an improvement in symptoms: In a double-blind study of 20 people with osteoarthritis, half of those who took 6 mg per day of boron for eight weeks reported less pain and joint swelling and better function than those who got a placebo (Fracp).

Boron is a plentiful mineral found in many fruits, vegetables, nuts and dried beans (and in wine, cider and beer). Although boron levels in food vary with the amount in the soil in which they are grown, people who eat a diet rich in fruits and vegetables most likely get enough boron.

How It's Used

There is no recommended dietary intake for boron. Some suggest 1 mg of boron per day. It is included in some multivitamins.

Expert Opinion

There is some evidence boron supplements could help with osteoarthritis symptoms. However, if you want to increase your boron levels – and overall health – spend your money on more fresh vegetables and fruits instead.

Cautions

! Boron appears safe, but one study showed doses of 3 mg per day – the amount often found in commercial supplements – raised estrogen levels, which could possibly increase cancer and other risks for some women (Nielson).

! You may already be getting boron in your multivitamin. So if you decide to experiment with boron, limit the total dosage to less than 3 mg per day.

BOSWELLIA (Boswellia serrata)

Boswellia serrata is a tree from Asia that yields oils, gum and other products when its bark is peeled away. It's also known as frankincense and sometimes called salai guggal. The gum has long been used in Indian ayurvedic medicine for arthritis and musculoskeletal pains. In animal and test tube studies, boswellia inhibits leukotriene synthesis, which contributes to inflammation (Ammon). However, the results have been mixed. A double-blind German study showed it didn't alter rheumatoid arthritis symptoms (Sander), but two studies of boswellia in combination with other herbs showed patients with both osteoarthritis and rheumatoid arthritis got relief from pain and inflammation (Chopra 1, Chopra 2). The other herbs were ginger, turmeric and ashwagandha (an Indian herb). A single-blind, placebo-controlled study found boswellia combined with turmeric and a zinc compound eased osteoarthritis pain and stiffness (Kulkarni).

How It's Used

Boswellia comes in a standardized extract of the gum oleoresin. A usual dosage is 150 mg three times a day for two to three months. It is also found in combination products.

This herb has a long tradition of use for arthritis in Asia and is generally safe, so it may be worth a try.

Caution
! Boswellia sometimes can cause diarrhea, nausea or a rash. Stop taking it if you have any side effects.

BROMELAIN *(Ananas comosus, or pineapple)*

Bromelain is a protein-digesting enzyme found in pineapple. A review of its reported uses include anti-inflammatory, blood-thinning and wound-healing (Taussig). It is sometimes recommended for sprains and strains, and several popular herb books recommend it to ease rheumatoid arthritis inflammation. However, there is no scientifically accepted evidence that bromelain relieves any arthritis symptoms.

There is some evidence for bromelain as an anti-inflammatory. In a 1981 study of rats with artificially induced arthritis, bromelain reduced inflammation better then several other drugs, including aspirin (Taussig). In an uncontrolled study from 1964, 29 people with moderate to severe arthritis (rheumatoid arthritis, osteoarthritis and gout) added bromelain to their glucocorticoid (steroid) therapy for one to 13 months. Overall, swelling decreased and mobility increased in 18, swelling increased in two, and there was little change in five. The one person with gout did not improve (Cohen).

How It's Used
Bromelain extract comes in capsules. Dosage has been quoted at 400–600 mg three times per day.

Expert Opinion
There's not enough evidence to say if this helps with any kind of arthritis.

Caution
! Bromelain can increase the effect of blood-thinning drugs, so it may cause bleeding if you are taking other blood-thinning herbs or drugs.

! It can enhance the effect of tetracycline antibiotics.

! Large doses can upset your stomach and cause cramps.

CARTILAGE

See Collagen

CAT'S CLAW *(Uncaria tomentosa)*

Cat's claw is a vine that grows wild in the Peruvian Amazon, where it has a long tradition as a treatment for inflammation and "bone pain." It gets its name, "uña de gato," from claw-shaped thorns. New research is promising: A 1998 animal study shows it does act as an anti-inflammatory and as an antioxidant to prevent inflammation and other cell damage (Sandoval-Chacon). It also may protect the gastrointestinal system from damage by NSAIDs. In the same study, rats who were given a cat's claw "tea" and injected with indomethacin (an NSAID) had nearly normal intestinal tracts compared to rats that didn't take the herb and had pronounced damage.

How It's Used

The usual dosage is 500–1,000 mg three times a day. Traditionally, the bark of the vine is boiled to make a tea. It's also sold as tea bags and ground up for capsules.

Expert Opinion

Although this herb is widely used in South America, there are at present no humans studies to show this herb works or that it is safe.

Cautions

❗ Cat's claw may increase the risk of bleeding if taken with other blood thinners.

Good Advice

• Be aware that there are two other plants called cat's claw, one of them poisonous. Check labels and sources carefully. The toxic cat's claw is a member of the acacia species and grows in the American southwest. Another cat's claw also comes from Peru but is *Uncaria guianensis*. The one tested is *Uncaria tomentosa*.

CAYENNE OR RED PEPPER *(Capsicum species)*

Red pepper can do more than spice up your food. It contains capsaicin, which prompts the release of endorphins, the body's natural pain-relievers. It is also thought to block pain by interfering with substance P, a chemical responsible for transmitting pain signals (Rains). It's most often used as a cream applied directly to the skin to give pain relief from both osteoarthritis and rheumatoid arthritis (McCarthy). Because the effect is temporary, you need to use capsaicin cream regularly to get relief. It produces a burning pain when you first start using it, and then eases discomfort.

How It's Used

You can find many creams with 0.025 to 0.075 percent capsaicin sold over-the-counter, or ask your doctor for a prescription for a more potent version. Apply directly to painful areas as directed.

Expert Opinion

This herbal remedy is recommended by the American College of Rheumatology as part of the treatment plan for osteoarthritis of the knee. Hot pepper may cool your pain, although large amounts taken internally can upset the stomach and the ointment may irritate your skin. Test on a small area first, and discontinue if it causes irritation.

Caution

! Don't use capsaicin cream on irritated or broken skin.

! Be sure to wash your hands carefully before touching your eyes or other body parts, and keep out of the reach of children. Pepper can damage delicate tissues. For the same reason, wash off all the cream *before* you shower or bathe.

! Don't use with a heat source, such as a heating pad.

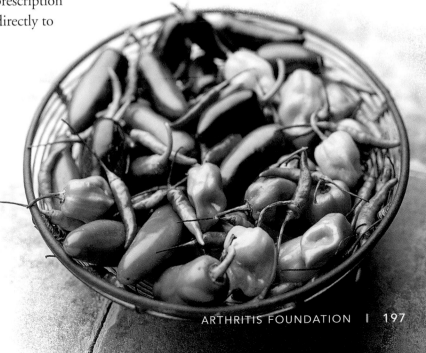

CHINESE HERBS

Herbs play a key role in traditional Chinese medicine (see page 33). They are used, along with other treatments, to help balance the body's vital life force, called qi (pronounced chee).

You've probably heard of ginseng (see page 216) and ginkgo (see page 215), but there are many more Asian herbs used to treat arthritis. One of the herbs, thunder god vine (*Tripterygium wilfordii*, page 228), shows promise in treating autoimmune diseases.

Chinese herbs aren't all herbs: Although most are from plants and vegetables, some are from minerals or animal products. They are most often used in combination formulas that contain two to two dozen or more ingredients, and are prepared as pills, potions and liniments. Teas or "soups" are made by boiling dried herbs in water to make a concentrated liquid.

The preparations are available in standardized formulations for many ills, or custom blended for individuals by the practitioner after making a diagnosis. There are too many of these combinations to discuss here, and many have not been studied outside of Asia. Some are beginning to be studied in the United States, with positive results. A randomized controlled study published in the *Journal of the American Medical Association* in 1998 showed that patients given either a standard or a customized blend of Chinese herbs for irritable bowel syndrome did much better than those on placebo (Bensoussan).

Expert Opinion

Chinese herbs follow centuries-old traditions and are aimed at balancing the body's functions and energy. They are often given along with acupuncture (see page 135). Some people say they have found significant relief from these herbs. However, because they are used in combinations, seek out an expert if you wish to try them.

Caution

! Be wary about the sources of Chinese herbs. Some grown in Asia may contain contaminants such as pesticides or heavy metals, and some preparations have been known to be mixed with steroids and other drugs. Consult a practitioner with experience diagnosing and prescribing, and with a reputable source for herbs.

! A product that contained dangerous drugs called "black pearls" was being marketed for a while.

CHONDROITIN SULFATE

See also Glucosamine

Chondroitin sulfate exists naturally in your cartilage. It's thought to draw fluid into the tissue to give cartilage elasticity and to slow cartilage breakdown by protecting it from destructive enzymes. As a supplement, it comes from cattle trachea and is often taken along with glucosamine to relieve osteoarthritis symptoms. It's been used in Europe for osteoarthritis pain for years.

Although it hasn't been proven to reverse cartilage loss, in some studies it appeared to help stop joint degeneration, improve function, and ease pain. In one placebo-controlled study, joint-narrowing in the knee was stabilized in some of those who took chondroitin (Uebelhart). Another controlled study looked at osteoarthritis of the finger joints for a period of three years. Among the group that took chondroitin, there was a significant decrease in the number of patients with new erosions in their finger joints (Verbruggen).

Chondroitin is a slow-acting supplement: It takes two months or more for the effects to show up. Some have questioned whether chondroition can be easily absorbed when taken orally. However, studies show it relieves arthritis symptoms.

How It's Used

The recommended dosage of chondroitin is 1,200 mg a day divided into two doses. It's most often taken in combination with glucosamine although there are no studies that show the two together are any more effective than either taken alone.

Expert Opinion

Because there are no serious side effects, it's worth a try. It doesn't seem to help everyone: If you have severe cartilage loss, you probably won't see any improvement. If you don't see any progress after two or three months, it may not work for you.

Cautions

! Occasional side effects include nausea and indigestion. However, it hasn't been studied over time, so effects of long-term use aren't known.

! It is molecularly quite similar to the blood thinner heparin, so be aware that it may increase your chances of bleeding if you are taking other drugs or herbs that are blood thinners.

! Some chondroitin supplements are made from shark cartilage, but this is not recommended as a source. The quality and amount of active ingredients varies, and some experts are concerned about possible heavy metal contamination.

CMO

(cetyl myristoleate; cerasomal-cis-9-cetylmyristoleate)

You'll see this supplement advertised in many places as a "cure" for just about every kind of arthritis, including osteoarthritis, rheumatoid arthritis, lupus, fibromyalgia, ankylosing spondylitis and more. Advertisements promise it can modify the immune system, and banish your arthritis permanently after only 10 to 20 days of treatment.

Although there is one promising animal study, there's no accepted scientific evidence so far that CMO can help with arthritis of any type. The hoopla is based on an intriguing 1993 study from the National Institutes of Health. In experiments to induce rheumatoid arthritis in mice, a researcher noted that Swiss albino mice seemed to be immune. He isolated cetyl myristoleate as the protective substance, and when it was injected into rats,

> Instructions for use of CMO advise you to stop taking your methotrexate. Don't do it! Methotrexate is proven to prevent joint damage.

they were also protected against arthritis (Diehl).

No human research has been published, so there is no accepted scientific evidence to show CMO is safe or effective.

However, the real concern about CMO is from instructions some vendors have been giving to people taking immunosuppressant or disease-modifying arthritis drugs such as glucocorticoids (steroids) and methotrexate. They say that these drugs interfere with CMO activity, and advise you to stop taking them before beginning CMO or they won't "guarantee" it will help you. Some vendors say you have to have stopped taking methotrexate for two years before taking CMO, others say two weeks. This is dangerous advice, because methotrexate and glucocorticoids prevent joint damage. In the weeks or years that you are waiting to see if an unproven remedy might help your arthritis, you could be sustaining irreversible joint damage.

The CMO sold as a dietary supplement comes from beef tallow. Similar waxy fatty acids are used in many processed foods such as chocolate, and in cosmetics. It's also sold to treat animals.

How It's Used

CMO capsules are taken daily for 10 to 20 days. People are told to discontinue steroids or methotrexate before taking this supplement; and to avoid alcohol, chocolate and caffeine while taking CMO.

Expert Opinion

Although the animal test is promising, there's no scientifically accepted evidence CMO will do anything for any kind of arthritis.

Cautions

! There's no clinical evidence that CMO is dangerous or safe.

! The real danger to your health could come if you stop taking prescribed medications for arthritis. Consult your doctor before discontinuing any prescribed medication.

COLLAGEN

You may have seen advertisements that say taking shark, chicken or cow cartilage in capsules or pills can help ease symptoms of both osteoarthritis and rheumatoid arthritis and contribute to "healthy joints." It sounds logical: If your cartilage is damaged, wouldn't supplements of animal cartilage help to repair it?

So far, the answer is no. There is no accepted scientific evidence that taking animal cartilage in supplements relieves symptoms of any type of arthritis. There's also no accepted evidence that gelatin products (a collagen-related substance) advertised "to rebuild cartilage" have any effect on arthritis.

However, research results of a specific collagen substance extracted from animal carti-lage is promising. Called type II collagen, it's being studied to treat rheumatoid and juvenile rheumatoid arthritis. It isn't expected to help repair or preserve your cartilage directly. Rather, it works to suppress the autoimmune response associated with rheumatoid arthritis that attacks healthy joints.

In several animal and human studies, type II collagen taken orally has reduced inflammation and pain for some with rheumatoid arthritis, with no or few side effects. A randomized, double-blind, placebo-controlled Harvard University study of 60 people with severe active rheumatoid arthritis found those who took small doses of type II chicken collagen for three months had a significant improvement in swollen and tender joints compared to those on placebo. Four people had a complete remission (Trentham). A larger study of 274 patients that looked at various doses found good results at the lowest dosage of 20 micrograms per day (Barnett).

Responses seem to vary with individuals or the source of collagen, and collagen did not do as well as methotrexate in one study. One study divided 90 people with early rheumatoid arthritis into three groups. One group got a placebo, the other two groups received type II collagen extracted from cow cartilage in doses of 1 mg per day or 10 mg per day. Researchers found no significant difference between the three groups. Four individuals, however, had very good responses (Sieper). When compared with methotrexate in a randomized, double-blind, placebo-controlled trial, people who took type II collagen instead of methotrexate worsened significantly during the study (Hauselmann).

A large-scale, multicenter trial of 772 people with active rheumatoid arthritis is underway now, sponsored by a company that is seeking FDA approval for a type II collagen product made from chicken sternums.

How It's Used

The type II collagen that has been found effective in studies has been given at very low doses of 500 micrograms or less. In the ongoing study, people are receiving doses of 60 micrograms. You may see ads that suggest much higher doses. Talk to your doctor about taking any kind of cartilage or collagen.

Expert Opinion

Type II collagen supplements are promising, but there isn't enough evidence to show they ease rheumatoid arthritis symptoms or that they do anything for osteoarthritis. It makes sense to wait for the results of a large study due in 2000. As for cartilage, there is no accepted scientific evidence that shark, cow or chicken cartilage supplements help with any arthritis symptoms.

Cautions

! Cartilage and collagen are not the same thing. Type II collagen, the material being studied, is a specific substance extracted from cartilage.

! Talk to your doctor before you try any cartilage or type II collagen supplements.

! Be careful with dosage: Small doses appear to be more effective.

! Read labels: Some "cartilage" products contain many kinds of herbs and other substances.

! There are no toxic side effects, but type II collagen at high doses may cause nausea in some people.

COPPER

Copper is an essential trace metal that helps in bone growth and may help prevent bone loss. Osteoporosis and bone abnormalities are associated with copper deficiency. Copper is also known to be an anti-inflammatory, and to boost the activity of NSAIDs without increasing risks of ulcers (JAMA).

For years, it's been suggested that supplements of copper could ease the aches of many kinds of arthritis by lowering inflammation. Folklore has it that wearing copper bracelets eases rheumatoid arthritis pain. Although some doctors have scoffed at this, a significant number of those wearing the copper bracelets in a controlled study said they got some relief (Walker). See Copper Bracelets, page 151.

Copper complexes have been used to treat a range of rheumatic diseases, mostly in Europe. A review of studies from 1940 to 1971 that involved 1,500 patients with different kinds of arthritis showed copper complexes helped some people with rheumatoid arthritis, ankylosing spondylitis, gout and Reiter's syndrome (Sorenson). However, the studies were uncontrolled. The copper complexes were given by injection or intravenously; and although many improved, not everyone benefited. Some complexes provoked side effects such as nausea, vomiting, diarrhea and anemia.

The role of copper in rheumatoid arthritis is complicated, and there isn't scientifically accepted evidence that oral supplements help. Copper deficiency is rare, and there is no established recommended dietary intake for copper. You can increase your copper intake through foods. Interestingly, a chocolate and nut treat might help: Foods high in copper include nuts, chocolate, seeds and dried beans.

How It's Used

The usual dosage is 1 mg to 3 mg per day of copper chelate. It's in many multivitamins, sometimes in doses of 2 mg.

Expert Opinion

There are uncontrolled studies that suggest copper may relieve arthritis symptoms. But the evidence for using copper to treat rheumatoid arthritis isn't conclusive. It's probably worth checking to see that you are getting a total daily intake of about 3 mg from varying sources (see Cautions). Wearing a copper bracelet won't hurt, but don't count on it to help, either.

! People who have Wilson's disease, a genetic disorder in which copper accumulates in the body, should never take copper supplements.

Good Advice
• Copper is in many multivitamins, and if you have copper plumbing in your pipes, you're getting copper in your drinking water, too. A supplement might give you an overdose.

CURCUMIN

See Turmeric

DEVIL'S CLAW (*Harpagophytum procumbens*)

This folk remedy comes from an African plant that is named for the bumpy hooks that cover its fruit. The roots contain harpagoside, which has anti-inflammatory and pain-killing properties. It is used in Africa for arthritic conditions and is a popular treatment for rheumatoid arthritis in Europe.

Scientific research results are mixed. A 1983 animal study showed that it didn't reduce swelling in rats even at doses 100 times or greater than the recommended daily dose for humans (Whitehouse). In a double-blind, placebo-controlled 1998 study of 118 patients with chronic low back pain, Devil's claw was found to relieve pain significantly better than the placebo (Chrubasik 2). However, the back pain was from undetermined causes and not necessarily arthritis.

Devil's claw is also used as a digestive stimulant.

How It's Used
Devil's claw comes as a tea, tincture and capsules. Look for the active ingredient, harpagoside, on the label. Some people take 2 to 10 grams per day of Devil's claw for rheumatoid arthritis.

Expert Opinion
Devil's claw appears to be safe, but there's no evidence it helps rheumatoid arthritis.

Caution

! Devil's claw is used to stimulate stomach acids, so be careful if you have gastric or duodenal ulcers or are taking other drugs that may irritate the intestines, such as NSAIDs.

! Don't take it if you are pregnant, as it might stimulate contractions.

DHEA (dehydroepiandrosterone)

DHEA, which is short for the tongue-twister dehydroepiandrosterone, is a mild androgen (male hormone) produced naturally in the body that is used to make many other hormones including the sex hormones testosterone and estrogen. It has been touted as a miracle cure for everything from cancer to old age. Studies have yet to prove most of these claims, but it shows promise as a lupus therapy. DHEA levels are low in those with lupus. In a multicenter trial of 191 women with mild to moderate lupus who were taking prednisone, 200 mg of DHEA per day relieved symptoms of pain, inflammation and fatigue and allowed them to reduce their daily glucocorticoid dose (van Vollenhoven, Petri). The women also said they felt better.

Since low DHEA levels are also found in those with rheumatoid arthritis and juvenile rheumatoid arthritis (Khalkhali-Ellis), it seems possible DHEA supplements could help with those conditions as well. But so far, this hasn't been scientifically shown. It's also been suggested for scleroderma, but again there is no evidence it can help.

It's not clear exactly how DHEA works to ease symptoms, but it's known that estrogen hormones can increase immune function whereas androgens suppress it, and that the estrogen-testosterone balance is off in women with lupus.

Products from wild yam are sometimes marketed as natural sources of DHEA, but they don't contain DHEA in any form your body can use (see Wild Yam, page 234). Although the raw material for DHEA supplements is extracted from wild yam, is has to be altered in a laboratory to be biologically available.

Also, products that claim to contain DHEA vary greatly in the amount and purity, so there's no way to ensure quality or the correct dosage.

How It's Used

If you want to try DHEA, ask your doctor to monitor you for a trial session, and to order DHEA that has been prepared by a compounding pharmacy so you can be sure you are getting a regulated amount of the real thing (see Resources). In an ongoing study, women are taking 200 mg per day, but your doctor might start with a much lower dosage.

Expert Opinion

DHEA could be the first new drug to be approved for lupus in decades and it shows promise in several other areas. However, it has risks, so don't try DHEA without a doctor's supervision.

Cautions

! This drug, like all hormones, can be dangerous. In the ongoing, multicenter study, researchers are finding that in some women DHEA reduces levels of HDL, the good cholesterol; and increases estrogen levels and, possibly, cancer risks. It also causes acne in some people.

! Don't self-prescribe and don't try DHEA off the shelf: The amount and purity of DHEA can vary widely.

! There is a possibility of liver damage if you're taking azathioprine (*Imuran*) or methotrexate. Also, liver cysts, certain brain tumors and sterility in men can be caused by testosterone and could possibly be a problem for people taking DHEA.

DMSO (dimethyl sulfoxide)

See also MSM (methyl sulfonyl methane)

This controversial chemical has been in and out of favor in the United States for the past 40 years. A by-product of wood processing, it's a chemical used in paint thinner and antifreeze. It also has many medical uses and is prescribed in other countries for a range of ailments including arthritis and related diseases. DMSO is applied externally to relieve joint and soft tissue inflammation, soften collagen and transport just about anything – including other drugs – across cell membranes. It's also given internally.

Back in the 1960s, it was being hailed as a new therapy for all kinds of arthritis, including scleroderma. But studies of DMSO were halted in the mid-'60s after very high doses damaged the lens of the eye in animal studies. (There have been no problems with eyes in human studies.) Today, it is widely used in Russia and other countries for rheumatoid arthritis and osteoarthritis. In the United

States, it is used by veterinarians for musculoskeletal problems in animals, and has FDA approval for use in humans for a bladder condition called interstitial cystitis. It isn't approved for other medical uses, but it's the chemical used to protect organs during the transplantation process, and to protect human tissue (such as bone marrow, stem cells and embryos) when frozen for storage.

DMSO has its advocates in the medical community. There's research that suggests it can relieve pain and increase function for those with arthritis (Eberhardt), and that it may ease finger ulcers in scleroderma and relieve blood vessel constrictions in Raynaud's (Scherbel). But DMSO research is mixed. It has a shady reputation in the United States because of those animal studies, and will need more research before it can be considered safe and effective.

MSM (methyl sulfonyl methane) is derived from DSMO and is now being promoted as a cure-all (see page 223).

How It's Used

DMSO is given orally, intravenously, injected and applied externally. It is important to use only medical-quality DMSO.

If you are interested in trying this, ask a doctor to help you find and use this product safely. There is a program for treatment at Oregon Health Sciences University in Portland, Oregon (see Resources).

RESOURCE ✳ DMSO

Stanley Jacob, MD
Gerlinger Professor, School of Medicine
Oregon Health Sciences University
3181 SW Sam Jackson Park Road
Portland, OR 97201-3098
Phone: 503/494-8474

Expert Opinion

Don't try this without a doctor's help. DMSO is commonly sold in industrial grades that are not suitable for human use, and it's not readily available in a purified form for medical use. Much of what you will find on the market is not chemically pure and can hurt you.

Caution

! Do not buy DMSO yourself. It may not be pure, and DMSO can be hazardous. Its ability to transport molecules across cell walls means any ingredients in it or on your skin are absorbed along with it. Impure products may cause skin irritation; kidney, liver and vision problems; and speed up joint deterioration.

! It can cause bad breath or a bad taste in the mouth (like garlic or onions).

! Some people may have an allergic reaction or skin irritation and itching.

ECHINACEA
(Echinacea purpurea, Echinacea angustifolia)

This native North American wildflower is one of the top-selling herbal products in Europe and the United States, taken by millions at the first sign of a sniffle. It's been touted as an immune system "booster," and a treatment for a variety of ills. In Germany, where it has been studied most, it's approved by the national health agency for upper respiratory infections, wounds and lower urinary tract infections.

However, United States experts say there isn't enough hard scientific evidence yet to prove the claims for echinacea. Although it has been widely studied, experts find much of the research is flawed. An analysis of published trials found none of good enough quality to be conclusive (Melchart). Experts do agree that echinacea shows much promise for treating infections and wounds, and no serious side effects have been reported in more than a century of use in Europe (O'Hara).

There's concern about what it may do to those with autoimmune diseases whose immune system is already overactive. Nobody really seems to know, and most experts advise those with rheumatoid arthritis, lupus or other autoimmune diseases to steer clear of echinacea.

How It's Used

Echinacea comes in capsules, tablets, extracts, tinctures and juices. It can also be made into a tea, but this isn't recommended because some of its active ingredients don't dissolve in water. The usual dose in capsules is 900 mg three times per day; in tincture, 15–30 drops two to five times per day.

Expert Opinion

There's some evidence echinacea can inhibit infections, but it hasn't been proven yet, and there's no evidence it helps any kind of arthritis. Taken at the onset of symptoms, it might help you recover from a cold faster. If you do have an autoimmune disease, don't take it.

Cautions

! Herbal experts advise against echinacea for those with severe illness and autoimmune diseases such as rheumatoid arthritis and lupus.

! It may interact with or intensify conventional drugs. One source warned not to take echinacea with methotrexate or other drugs that affect the liver as it might contribute to liver damage.

! Do not take with corticosteroids or other immunosuppressing drugs (Miller).

! Don't take echinacea daily for longer than eight weeks. A course of 10–14 days is best.

ELEUTHERO

See Ginseng

EVENING PRIMROSE OIL

See GLA (gamma linolenic acids)

FISH OIL

See also gamma linolenic acids, flaxseed

Oils from cold water fish such as salmon and mackerel show promise for relieving arthritis symptoms. More than 18 studies have shown fish oil reduces inflammation and pain for those with rheumatoid arthritis. In one study of those with Raynaud's, it improved tolerance to cold.

Fish oil contains the omega-3 fatty acids eicosapentaenoic acid (EPA) and docosahexaenoic acid (DHA) that help you maintain a healthy nervous system, cell walls and vision. These fatty acids also appear to ease arthritis symptoms by providing the building blocks for anti-inflammatory agents.

In one double-blind, placebo-controlled study of 64 patients with stable rheumatoid arthritis who were taking either fish oil or a placebo, participants in the group taking fish oil were able to significantly reduce their NSAID use (Lau). In a similar study, those taking fish oil had a decrease in tender joints and other symptoms, and some were able to discontinue NSAID use completely without having a flare (Kremer).

Fish oil also seems to improve Raynaud's phenomenon. In a study of 32 people with primary or secondary Raynaud's who took fish oil or a placebo, there was a significant improvement in reactions to cold temperatures in the fish oil group (DiGiacomo). EPA and DHA have also been shown to improve heart health by thinning blood and lowering triglycerides, and nutritionists also think they help prevent some kinds of cancer.

How It's Used

The usual dose is about 3 grams (3,000 mg) total of EPA/DHA. Because fish oil sold as a dietary supplement comes in capsules with varying percentages of EPA and DHA, you may have to take between 10 and 15 capsules a day. There are higher potency pills. Look on the label for the amount of EPA/DHA. If it doesn't say how much, don't buy that brand. If you aren't sure of the math, ask a pharmacist to help you so you get the right dosage.

Expert Opinion

Fish oil has a good record for easing rheumatoid arthritis inflammation and may help with Raynaud's, but you have to swallow a lot of pills. You can get some of these benefits by eating cold water fish such as salmon three times a week (see Change Your Oil, page 170). Also, flaxseed contains another helpful fatty acid that has the building blocks for EPA (see Flaxseed, page 211).

Cautions

! If you decide to try fish oil supplements, be sure to tell your doctor. Fish oil thins the blood, which means it can multiply the effects of any other blood thinners you are taking (including NSAIDs and herbs such as garlic and turmeric).

Good Advice

- Be careful with the old standby, cod liver oil. It is rich in vitamins A and D and you might overdose on those vitamins.

FLAXSEED *(Linum usitatissimum)*

See also Fish Oil, Gamma Linolenic Acids

This plant-based oil is believed by some to be next best to fish oil for arthritis, but so far there aren't any good studies that prove this. The belief it may reduce inflammation in rheumatoid arthritis comes from its composition and studies that show it can increase EPA levels. Like many vegetable oils, it contains linoleic acid. But it also contains an omega-3 oil called alpha linolenic acid that can be converted into EPA – the fish oil ingredient that reduces inflammation in rheumatoid arthritis and may ease Raynaud's symptoms. Flaxseed contains the most building blocks for EPA of any plant oil.

The one study that looked at flaxseed oil and rheumatoid arthritis wasn't very promising (Nordstrom). In a placebo-controlled trial of 22 people, the group taking flaxseed oil for three months showed some blood-thinning but no improvement in rheumatoid arthritis symptoms. However, it may be that the complete diet of those in the study affected the outcome: Flaxseed oil is better converted into anti-inflammatory EPA when linoleic acids from other vegetable oils are restricted.

In another randomized, controlled trial, one group ate a diet high in flaxseed oil and low in linoleic acids. The other group ate a typical Western diet. After the initial four-week period, both groups supplemented their diets with fish oil for four weeks. Researchers found flaxseed oil raised the EPA levels about the same amount as did fish oil supplements (Mantzioris).

It's also possible flaxseed will help with lupus. In a small uncontrolled study of nine people with lupus nephritis, 30 grams of flaxseed a day significantly lowered cholesterol, thinned blood, reduced inflammation and improved kidney function (Clark).

How It's Used

Flaxseed is available as an oil, and in capsules, meal and flour. Because flaxseed doesn't contain EPA but only the materials to make it, it takes more flaxseed to equal the amount in fish oil. However, the oil can be used in salad dressings and for low-temperature cooking, which increases intake. Also, you can cook with flaxseed and flaxseed meal. These can be sprinkled on cereals or baked into just about anything. Some sources recommend taking 1 to 3 tablespoons a day of the oil or about

30 grams (one-fourth of a cup) of the meal. See Resources for where to get recipes.

Expert Opinion

There is mixed evidence that flaxseed can ease arthritis symptoms, but good evidence that it contains ingredients that do act as anti-inflammatories. Flaxseed has no side effects, and may have other benefits. It contains lignans, which are believed to reduce growth of both breast and colon cancer tumors. The meal also helps prevent constipation.

Cautions

! There are no known adverse effects, but some people experience gas or loose bowels. Start with smaller amounts and build up to the recommended dosage.

GAMMA LINOLENIC ACID
(GLA; evening primrose oil and borage oil)

See also Fish Oil, Flaxseed

These common weedy plants contain the essential fatty acid gamma linolenic acid (GLA), also found in black currant seed oils. GLA is an omega-6 fatty acid converted by the body to make anti-inflammatory agents. Although evening primrose oil may be better known, borage oil has a higher percentage of GLA.

Several studies show that GLA supplements can relieve rheumatoid arthritis pain and inflammation. When people with rheumatoid arthritis were given either evening primrose oil, evening primrose oil and fish oil, or a placebo for a year, both groups taking evening primrose oil did better than placebo (Belch). All three groups were able to reduce their NSAID dosages: 73 percent of those taking evening primrose oil alone; 80 percent of those taking evening primrose oil and fish oil together; 33 percent of those in the placebo group.

In another controlled study using borage oil, 37 people with rheumatoid arthritis were given either GLA or cotton seed oil. The group getting the GLA supplements showed clinically important relief of joint swelling and tenderness, but the placebo group showed no significant improvement (Leventhal).

Some folklore recommends rubbing these oils on your aching joints, or on the hands for those with Raynaud's. However, there's no evidence to support the external use of these oils.

How It's Used

The usual dosage is about 1.8 grams (1,800 mg) of GLA a day. Borage and evening primrose oils are only part GLA: To get that amount, you have to take a lot of borage oil and a *lot* more evening primrose oil. Check the ingredients on the label and see how much GLA is in a product. If it doesn't say, don't buy it. If you are taking borage oil, you will most likely need to take seven or eight 1,000-mg capsules that contain 240 mg of GLA a day. To get the same amount from evening primrose oil, you may need 40 capsules of 45-mg of GLA each. Look for high dosage capsules, and be prepared to do some math. If you aren't sure of the math, ask a pharmacist to help you.

Expert Opinion

GLA oils have been shown to reduce rheumatoid arthritis inflammation, and are worth a try. However, not all of the omega-6 fatty acids from evening primrose oil or borage oil end up as GLA: Some are converted into arachidonic acid, which provides the chemicals for prostaglandins and leukotrienes that cause inflammation. These oils are also expensive, and not covered by insurance. You can improve your health – and possibly arthritis – by improving the balance of oils in your diet (see Change Your Oil, page 170).

Cautions

! If you decide to try GLA supplements, be sure to tell your doctor. These thin the blood, which means they can multiply the effects of any other blood thinners you are taking (including NSAIDs and herbs such as ginger and turmeric).

GIN-SOAKED RAISINS

This modern folk remedy of a handful of raisins soaked in gin is supposed to ease arthritis aches. If it does, it might be the gin dulling the pain. Grapes and raisins do contain anti-inflammatories, but it takes more than a handful to get an effect.

How It's Used

Add raisins to your breakfast cereal or to salads, or eat them as snacks. Drink grape juice. Skip the gin.

Expert Opinion

Grapes contain many beneficial vitamins, but it would take a lot of grapes or raisins to get any benefit.

Caution

! Alcoholic drinks, such as gin, are not recommended as a medical treatment. Heavy alcohol use can make your symptoms worse by depleting your body of nutrients and vitamins, and contributing to depression.

GINGER *(Zingiber officinale)*

The root of this beautiful lily is a staple in Asian cooking, and has been used most often to settle an upset stomach. It is used in both Chinese and ayurvedic medicine.

Laboratory research shows ginger is an anti-inflammatory and potentially a painkiller. It inhibits production of prostaglandins and leukotrienes, which cause pain and swelling. In an uncontrolled study of the effect of ginger on arthritis and muscle pain, all patients with musculoskeletal pain found some relief, and three-fourths of those with either rheumatoid arthritis or osteoarthritis had relief from pain and swelling (Srivastava). A randomized, controlled study of an Indian herbal remedy that combined ginger with boswellia, turmeric and ashwagandha showed similar results on people with both osteoarthritis and rheumatoid arthritis (Chopra 1, Chopra 2).

How It's Used

A tea made from one teaspoon of fresh grated ginger steeped in a cup of water may ease pain. Or take powdered ginger in capsules or tablets, or in a tincture. A hot compress that includes ginger root might ease aching joints. You can also increase your intake by using it generously in cooking. (Hint: Freeze fresh ginger root to make it easier to grate.)

Expert Opinion

Ginger may be worth a try for pain, and it may pep you up as well. It's long been used as an energizing tonic.

Caution

! In very large doses, ginger can have some of the same gastrointestinal effects as NSAIDs.

! It can increase bleeding risks if you are taking blood-thinning medications.

GINKGO (Ginkgo biloba)

You've probably heard of this herb as a treatment to improve memory. It comes from the leaves of the ginkgo, the world's oldest living species of tree. Scientists don't fully understand how ginkgo works, but believe its effects come from the combined action of all its chemical ingredients (O'Hara). Studies show ginkgo might improve memory and dementia by improving circulation, especially in capillaries, the smallest of blood vessels. A controlled German study showed it significantly increased the blood flow in finger capillaries (Jung), so it may also ease symptoms of Raynaud's by increasing circulation in hands and feet. It's used in Europe to treat Raynaud's.

How It's Used

A usual dosage is 120–160 mg per day of *Ginkgo biloba* standardized to 6 percent terpene lactones and 24 percent flavone glycosides. It may take six to nine weeks before you notice an effect.

Expert Opinion

Ginkgo biloba may help with memory loss, but so far there is no scientific proof it eases Raynaud's. However, there is a very low risk of side effects.

Cautions

! Ginkgo may increase the risk

of bleeding if you are also taking blood-thinning drugs.

! There are few side effects, but a mild headache or an upset stomach is possible.

! Ginko seeds are used in Chinese medicine to treat asthma and coughing. They are mildly toxic and should be used with care.

GINSENG
American ginseng: *Panax quinquefolius*
Asian ginseng: *Panax ginseng*
Siberian ginseng: *Eleutherococcus senticosus*

Ginseng has been promoted for centuries as a tonic to reduce fatigue, improve performance, boost sex drive and fight cancer. It's one of the most popular and expensive herbs in the world, taken by millions. There is no evidence it can help with arthritis, but it may offer some benefit as an energy booster.

Ginseng is actually two different plant types. The *Panax* genus are related. These are *Panax ginseng*, the Asian ginseng; and *Panax quinquefolius*, the American ginseng. The Asian variety is the one used in most products. Siberian ginseng (*Eleutherococcus senticosus)* is of the same family and many similar claims are made for it. It's commonly called eleuthero.

Animal and test tube studies suggest both types of ginseng can benefit the immune and endocrine systems, but stud-ies on humans have shown conflicting results (O'Hara). In some studies, the *Panax* ginsengs have been shown to improve mental processing and attention (D'Angelo), although other studies didn't show this. Mice given one of four different kinds of ginseng preparations showed no difference in stamina or longevity compared to those given a placebo (Lewis). In another study, eleuthero ginseng did not improve stamina or energy for highly trained athletes (Dowling), and there are no human studies to support other claims.

How It's Used

Ginseng is usually taken in capsules or tablets, although it is also available as a tea. Ginseng dosage varies, but is usually about 100 mg standardized extract twice a day. Powered root dosage is usually

500–1,000 mg per day. To get good quality, look for products with a standardized ginsenoside content.

Expert Opinion

Ginseng itself is generally safe and can act as a mild stimulant. It may have other benefits as well, but this is not proven. The quality of ginseng products varies widely so you may be paying a big price (up to $20 an ounce) for something of little value – or that may do no more for you than a cup of coffee.

Cautions

Panax ginsengs may increase the effects of glucocorticoids, so those taking prednisone or other steroids shouldn't take ginseng.

! It can change your blood glucose levels, so those with juvenile onset diabetes should use it cautiously.

! It may increase the effects of estrogen drugs, blood thinners such as warfarin or other herbs with these qualities.

! Headaches and other bad reactions have been reported when taken with MAO inhibitors.

GLUCOSAMINE

See also Chondroitin

This supplement has been touted as an arthritis "cure," and although that's an overstatement it does appear to help ease the pain and stiffness of osteoarthritis. Glucosamine is a natural substance that provides the building blocks for the body to make and repair cartilage. The supplement is extracted from crab, lobster or shrimp shells, and taken in capsules. It's been used for a decade in Europe, and on animals in the United States for even longer.

There's a growing body of evidence that shows glucosamine eases osteoarthritis pain as well as NSAIDs. A 1998 double-blind study of 178 patients with osteoarthritis of the knee compared a daily dose of 1,500 mg of glucosamine sulfate with 1,200 mg of ibuprofen for four weeks. Both treatments relieved osteoarthritis symptoms, but the glucosamine group had significantly fewer side effects (Qiu). An analysis of English-language studies from 1975-1997 came to the same conclusion (da Camara), saying in some cases glucosamine performs as well as ibuprofen.

There's speculation it may rebuild cartilage, but no evidence yet. The National Institutes of Health is sponsoring a large

RESOURCE ✳
GLUCOSAMINE

Jason Theodasakis, MD, has a Web site that summarizes current medical research on these supplements: http://www.drtheo.com

study that should give some better answers in a few years.

You have to take glucosamine for about two months before you see any effects. It doesn't help everyone, so if you don't notice any changes after two months, it probably isn't working for you. If you have severe cartilage loss, it won't help you. It's not inexpensive: A day's dosage costs $0.80–$1.30, so comparison shop for the best value.

Glucosamine is sold as a "sulfate" and as a "hydrochloride." Experts say both perform equally well. It's often sold and taken with chondroitin, another material needed for healthy cartilage, but there are no studies that show the combination works better than taking either alone (Kelly).

How It's Used

Glucosamine comes in capsules and a drink, and also a cream. The usual dosage is 1,500 mg per day taken in two doses (2,000 mg for those who weigh 200 pounds or more). It's often combined with chondroitin, another supplement believed to nourish cartilage. Look carefully at the labels. Some glucosamine products have added ingredients, such as vitamins or minerals, that you may not want. There's no evidence that the cream or any other topical application of glucosamine has any effect on osteoarthritis.

Expert Opinion

Some doctors are recommending this supplement, and even taking it themselves for osteoarthritis. Because it has no known serious side effects, it's worth a try. Some have found it can help reduce the need for pain-killers.

Cautions

! Side effects are occasional cases of indigestion or nausea. If that happens, you may want to try a different brand. However, the long-term effects of this supplement haven't been studied.

! Some vendors say not to take glucosamine if you have a shellfish allergy, although it is unlikely it will cause a reaction.

GREEN TEA (*Camellia sinensis*)

Green tea has received a lot of attention in recent years as a possible preventive for cancer and other chronic diseases (Weisburger). Now animal studies suggest it may also be useful in treating and preventing rheumatoid arthritis.

Green tea contains polyphenols, antioxidant compounds that have been shown to reduce inflammation and protect against cancer. It's been used medicinally in Asia for thousands of years. In Japan, drinking green tea is accepted as a cancer preventive (Fujiki), and in China the Shanghai Institute reported those who drink green tea have a lower risk of esophageal cancer. It may also help protect against heart disease.

An animal study looked at the effect of green tea on arthritis. Mice given extracts of green tea polyphenols had a significantly lower rate of arthritis than mice who were not given the green tea extracts. Those that did develop arthritis had mild cases (Haqqi).

More research is needed to see if green tea will have the same effect on humans. However, green tea doesn't appear to have any side effects, even in those who took 15 green tea capsules a day for six months (Fujiki).

How It's Used

Green tea is available loose and in bags for brewing, and is sold as an extract in capsules, tablets and tinctures. Based on animal studies, a suggested dosage would be 3 or 4 cups per day, or the equivalent of green tea extract. Some people take much more. A typical cup of tea has about 200 mg of polyphenols, so check the labels of green tea extract to see how much polyphenol each capsule contains. Don't take green tea with milk, as milk may interfere with the action of polyphenols.

Expert Opinion

The evidence isn't in yet to prove green tea can help rheumatoid arthritis, but the results of animal experiments are promising. Because green tea is generally safe, even in large amounts, it may be worth a try. You could substitute it for coffee, because green tea does contain caffeine.

Cautions

! Green tea might cause an allergic reaction in people with green tea asthma.

! If you have been told to limit caffeine intake, check with your doctor before deciding to drink large amounts of green tea. Some types are decaffeinated.

GUAIFENESIN

An ingredient found in many cough syrups and decongestants has garnered a gathering of those who say it will "cure" fibromyalgia and even ease rheumatoid arthritis symptoms. People who have been taking cold medicines with guaifenesin say their symptoms are much reduced or even disappear. The word-of-mouth theory is that fibromyalgia is due to a buildup of phosphate in the cells, which results in depleted energy. Guaifenesin supposedly gets rid of the excess phosphate.

However, there are no studies so far to show any evidence of either this disease theory or the effect of guaifenesin on fibromyalgia. An unpublished, double-blind study done at the Oregon Health Sciences University found no differences between women taking guaifenesin and those taking a placebo. The study, by fibromyalgia specialist Robert Bennett, MD, was funded by the National Fibromyalgia Research Foundation of Salem, Oregon.

You can read the Oregon Health Sciences University report on the Internet at http://www.myalgia.com. Enter the search term "guaifenesin" at the site.

How It's Used

Not recommended.

Expert Opinion

If you have a cold or a cough, this may be useful for thinning mucus buildup. But there's no hard evidence it's worth taking for fibromyalgia.

Cautions

! Be careful taking drugs for conditions other than indicated. Those with gout or kidney stones could experience an increase in symptoms because guaifenesin mobilizes uric acid in the body.

KAVA KAVA (*Piper methysticum*)

A relaxing, nonalcoholic drink made from the root of the kava has been a traditional social and ceremonial offering throughout the Pacific Islands for centuries (Norton). Now it's become a popular way to unwind in the West.

Studies show kava does work as a relaxant. It contains kava-lactones that may relieve anxiety, promote muscle relaxation and ease pain. In a randomized, double-blind controlled study from Germany, a kava extract significantly reduced anxiety compared to a placebo, with no side effects (Kinzler).

How It's Used

The usual daily dosage is 140–210 mg of kava-lactones in capsules. If you have a source of fresh kava and want to take it as a drink, the usual dose is 1 to 3 ml fresh kava.

Expert Opinion

Kava may enhance pain control by helping you relax.

Caution

! Take care not to mix with tranquilizers, other depression drugs or alcohol: They multiply kava's effects (Jamieson).

MAGNESIUM

Magnesium is a mineral needed for healthy tissue and bone, and supplements are often used to treat heart disease and other conditions. Chronic fatigue symptoms are connected with low magnesium levels and supplements have been shown to significantly improve pain, fatigue and other symptoms (Cox). It's in many nuts, grains and whole foods, but you may not get enough if you mostly eat processed foods.

Magnesium has also helped relieve fibromyalgia symptoms. A placebo-controlled study that looked at magnesium combined with malic acid in 24 women with fibromyalgia found fairly high doses eased pain and boosted energy (Russell).

How It's Used

Magnesium comes in many forms. For fibromyalgia, the *Fibromyalgia Wellness Letter* suggests the following amounts, divided into several doses and taken daily: malic acid, 1,200–2,400 mg; magnesium, 300–600 mg.

Expert Opinion

Some doctors recommend this supplement. Check with your doctor before trying it.

Cautions

! Magnesium can interact with blood pressure medication, so check with your doctor if you are taking any of those drugs.

! High doses of magnesium (more than 6 grams per day) can be toxic, because your body can't eliminate it.

! Don't take magnesium if you have kidney problems because you may not be able to process it properly.

! It may cause diarrhea or loose stools, especially when combined with malic acid. Remember milk-of-magnesia, the old standby laxative? Loose stools may be a sign to lower your dosage.

MELATONIN

Melatonin is a natural hormone that regulates your biological clock: It controls your sleep/wake cycle and helps regulate reproductive hormones. It's made in the pineal gland located deep in the brain, and our bodies make less of it as we age. Over the past few years, it's been widely marketed as a "miracle drug" supposed to slow aging, boost the immune system and cure sleep and sex problems. Although most of those claims haven't been proven, melatonin does appear to boost the immune system, and it does help regulate sleep. Studies show that in healthy adults, melatonin shortens the time needed to fall asleep and improves sleep quality. Shift workers and international travelers use it to help them adjust to time changes; people with insomnia and the elderly use it to improve sleep.

Because fibromyalgia is connected with sleep disturbances, it seems logical that melatonin could help. But research on its role in fibromyalgia has produced conflicting results. Studies have shown that women with fibromyalgia have too much melatonin (Korszun), not enough melatonin (Wikner), and the same amount of melatonin as women without fibromyalgia (Press). A study presented at the 1998 American College of Rheumatology meeting showed women with fibromyalgia slept better after a nightly dose of 2 mg of melatonin (Csuka).

Researchers agree more studies are needed on the relationship between melatonin and fibromyalgia. They are also advising those with autoimmune diseases not use melatonin. Specialists say those with lupus in particular should not take it.

How It's Used

The usual dose is 1 to 3 mg taken a few hours before bedtime.

Expert Opinion

Melatonin may be safe for people without any medical conditions, but its effects on those with autoimmune diseases or fibromyalgia aren't really known. So use with care. Talk to your doctor before you take it.

Cautions

! Melatonin is a hormone, and thus can have far-reaching and unpredictable effects. It's tightly regulated in the United Kingdom and other countries.

! Melatonin is not recommended for anyone with an autoimmune disease such as lupus, or for those with depression.

MSM (methyl sulfonyl methane)

See also DMSO

This supplement is being touted on the Internet as one of the newest "cures" for arthritis, and just about everything else from allergies to constipation. But so far, there's no scientific evidence to prove this. MSM is a sulfur compound formed in the breakdown of DMSO. It also is found in fresh fruits and vegetables, milk, fish and grains. It's destroyed when foods are processed, so those who mainly eat processed food may have low levels.

The same doctor who promoted DMSO developed MSM. He says MSM has many of the same anti-inflammatory qualities of

RESOURCE ✳ MSM

Stanley Jacob, MD
Gerlinger Professor,
    School of Medicine
Oregon Health Sciences University
3181 SW Sam Jackson Park Road
Portland, OR 97201-3098
Phone: 503/494-8474

DMSO and is safe. Some case reports and animal studies are interesting. In one mouse study, MSM eased rheumatoid arthritis-like effects (Moore). In another study, it reduced deaths from lupus nephritis in mice (Morton). There are no published human trials.

How It's Used

MSM is available in capsules and as a lotion from many sources.

Expert Opinion

There are no scientific studies of its effect on humans to show if it's safe, effective or worth trying.

Cautions

! MSM is supposed to be non-toxic, but there's no research that shows it's safe.

! Because it is made from DMSO, it's only as pure as the DMSO is, so be sure to get it from a reliable source.

SAM (S-adenosylmethionine)

See also Folic Acid

SAM is a naturally occurring compound produced from methionine, a sulfur-containing amino acid, and adenosine triphosphate (ATP). It's believed to improve joint mobility and relieve pain by boosting levels of ATP and supporting cartilage production. It's also reported to be an antidepressant and to prevent liver damage.

Marketed as a supplement for osteoarthritis in Europe for some time, it's now available in the United States under several brand names, most commonly called SAMe.

Double-blind clinical trials have shown SAM relieves osteoarthritis pain and other symptoms about as well as NSAIDs such as ibuprofen – and without the side effects (Muller-Fassbender). A double-blind, placebo-controlled study that used injections and tablets of SAM looked at its effect in those with mild and severe osteoarthritis. Overall, it was better than placebo, and the group with mild osteoarthritis had significantly greater pain relief than the controls (Bradley).

An analysis of controlled clinical studies of SAM used for depression found it was as effective as standard tricyclic antidepressants and better than placebo, with few side effects (Bressa). An open study looked at 195 patients who were given 400 mg of SAM for 15 days. The participants found their depression symptoms improved after both the seven-day and 15-day follow-up visits (Fava).

How It's Used

In studies, SAM was taken in doses of 200 mg to 400 mg three times per day. Folic acid is needed to make SAM, and many people do not get enough folic acid. Boosting your folic acid levels by eating dark leafy green vegetables may help natural SAM production.

Expert Opinion

SAM is a promising therapy that's worth a try for pain relief. More scientific evidence that it supports cartilage repair is needed.

Cautions

SAM may occasionally cause nausea or digestive upset, especially in large doses.

ST. JOHN'S WORT (Hypericum perforatum)

Most everyone has heard of this "natural *Prozac*": Widely prescribed by doctors in Europe (Ernst), it has become one of the top-selling herbal remedies in the United States as well. In fact, there are entire books written about the benefits of the hardy herb.

St. John's wort is a small yellow flower that grows wild throughout Europe and the United States, especially in northern California and Oregon. It's been used for thousands of years for a variety of conditions, including depression. Although it isn't known exactly how St. John's wort works, it contains the chemicals hypericin and hyperforin, and appears to act as an antidepressant by raising levels of serotonin. Serotonin levels are known to be low in people who are depressed and in those with fibromyalgia. St. John's wort may also have anti-inflammatory effects.

Many studies have shown it can relieve mild depression. A 1996 analysis of two dozen controlled clinical trials found it more effective than placebo for mild to moderate depression (O'Hara). More trials are needed to determine the long-term effects and best dosage for depression. A large-scale, three-year study funded by the NIH comparing St. John's wort with antidepressant drugs is in progress now.

How It's Used

St. John's wort comes in pills and a tincture. The dose used in some clinical trials is 300 mg three times a day of an extract standardized to 0.3 percent hypericin.

Expert Opinion

This herb may help with mild depression

and insomnia, but is not for serious depression. Like prescription drugs that increase serotonin (such as *Prozac*), you need to take it for several weeks before you feel an effect.

Cautions

! Don't take St. John's wort with other antidepressants or with alcohol: It can increase the effects.

! It may increase sensitivity to sunlight and risk of sunburn in fair-skinned people. People with lupus should not take it.

! Don't take St. John's wort if you are also taking other drugs that increase sun sensitivity.

! If you are very depressed, or if your symptoms don't improve after two months of treatment, talk to your doctor about a stronger antidepressant.

SELENIUM

Selenium is an essential mineral that protects cells from oxidation damage. Selenium levels are known to be low in people with rheumatoid arthritis and other inflammatory conditions (Tarp). In an animal study, mice with a lupus-like disease who were fed selenium survived significantly longer than the controls (O'Dell). However, there are no human studies that show selenium supplements alone can improve the symptoms.

A double-blind, placebo-controlled German study of 70 people with rheumatoid arthritis showed that those who took selenium supplements had fewer tender joints, less swelling and less morning stiffness at the end of six months (Heinle). But both groups were also getting fish oil supplements.

How It's Used

A usual dose is 50–200 micrograms. Doses of 900 micrograms have been shown to be toxic.

Expert Opinion

Selenium might be worth trying, but the human body requires only a very small amount of selenium. It can be toxic in larger doses, and and it's already in many multivitamins.

Cautions

! Selenium supplements should be taken only in tiny doses, and only after checking with your doctor. Check your multivitamin to see if you are already taking selenium.

STINGING NETTLE (*Urtica dioica*)

Folklore has it that "stinging" yourself with this irritating weed on your painful joints can ease rheumatoid arthritis flares. The practice, called "urtication," is said to reduce swelling and pain in sore joints. Herbalists say the tiny stingers of the plant inject minute amounts of chemicals that cause the painful stinging sensation, but also may trigger anti-inflammatory reactions. So far, there is no scientific evidence to back up these claims.

Stinging nettle is more commonly taken internally, as an extract or by eating the cooked leaves. They are eaten as a delicacy in some areas. They contain boron (see page 193), which some believe may be helpful for both osteoarthritis and rheumatoid arthritis pain. In test tube studies, nettle leaf extract has been shown to inhibit chemicals that cause inflammation (Obertreis).

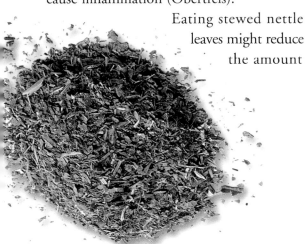

Eating stewed nettle leaves might reduce the amount of anti-inflammatory drugs needed for pain relief. A 1997 open, randomized German study compared the effects of 200 mg of diclofenac (an NSAID) with a 50-mg dose given along with stewed nettles in 40 people with osteoarthritis. Those taking the nettle leaf along with one-fourth the usual dosage of diclofenac did just as well as those taking the full dosage of diclofenac. Pain, stiffness, function and protein serum levels in both groups improved about 70 percent (Chrubasik).

How It's Used

Nettle extract is sold in capsules. To determine if it is helping relieve your symptoms, begin taking it along with your usual NSAID dosage. Decrease your NSAID dosage slowly as long as you get pain relief. If the pain returns, increase your NSAID dosage slightly until you get relief again.

If you want to try "stinging" away your pain or eating the leaves, you may have to grow your own nettle to get fresh leaves. Use gloves to pick the nettles. If using externally, try "stinging" one area at a time: It smarts. To eat, steam the fresh leaves and serve as a vegetable. They lose their "sting" when cooked.

Expert Opinion

Taken as a supplement or eaten, nettle

may boost the effects of anti-inflammatory drugs. Used externally, it could be that the pain from "stings" may override your aches rather than ease them.

Cautions

! Taken internally, cooked nettles have no known side effects.

! An allergic reaction is possible.

THUNDER GOD VINE (*Tripterygium wilfordii*)

See also Chinese Herbs

This vinelike plant has been used in many forms to treat autoimmune diseases in China and is now drawing Western interest. Most information has been based on personal anecdotes or clinical experience (what doctors observe). But there have been some test tube and animal studies that show it can interfere with the production of chemicals responsible for immune responses and inflammation (Lipsky).

Another study (Chou) compared thunder god vine with four Chinese herbal formulas used to treat acute arthritis or autoimmune diseases. The results of the test tube study showed that small amounts of thunder god vine extract alone inhibited the release of pain chemicals as well as several times as much of the formulas.

How It's Used

The active ingredient is found in the roots of the plant. Extracts were used in the studies, but no standard dose for humans has been established.

Expert Opinion

The uncontrolled clinical evidence looks promising. It's not enough, however, to show thunder god vine is safe or effective. Controlled studies are needed.

Cautions

! Leaves and flowers of this plant are highly toxic and can cause death. Be sure any preparation is made from the root only.

! Dose-related side effects include mouth dryness, loss of appetite, nausea and rash.

TURMERIC
(*Curcuma longa, Curcuma domestica*)

A root related to ginger, turmeric has traditionally been used in Indian ayurvedic medicine to treat clogged arteries, inflammation, bruises, bursitis and other ills. It's used lavishly in Indian cooking, especially in curries, for flavor and to add color. Turmeric is also used in traditional Chinese medicine formulations to treat arthritic pain.

Curcumin is the active ingredient. When combined with other ingredients such as boswellia and zinc, it's been shown in test tube and animal research to inhibit prostaglandins and to stimulate the production of cortisol. Both of these chemical actions might relieve inflammation (Kulkarni). Used with capsaicin, it relieved inflammation in rats with induced arthritis (Joe).

Two randomized controlled studies that looked at an herbal product that combined turmeric with boswellia, ginger and aswangandha found it relieved both pain and inflammation in rheumatoid arthritis and relieved pain in osteoarthritis (Chopra 1, Chopra 2).

How It's Used

The usual dose is 400 mg of turmeric three times per day in capsules or tablets. Or you can spice up your food with it.

Expert Opinion

The scientific evidence isn't complete, but it could provide some relief.

Cautions

! Turmeric is a food spice with no known side effects.

! Don't use turmeric if you have gallstones.

! Do not use during pregnancy.

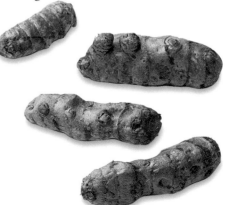

VALERIAN (*Valeriana officinalis*)

Valerian is a pink flower that grows wild throughout the Americas, Europe and Asia. Its root has been a popular treatment for insomnia and anxiety for centuries, and there are several studies that show it might be a effective and safe alternative to addictive sleep drugs. It's approved by German health officials as a mild sleep aid and sedative (O'Hara).

In one study, 128 people rated their sleep quality after taking one of three products: an over-the-counter product of valerian mixed with other ingredients, valerian alone, or a placebo. The valerian was rated significantly higher than placebo or the over-the-counter product by the participants who said it helped them fall asleep faster and sleep better. And it was most effective for those who had the most sleep problems (Leathwood).

There are no known serious side effects, and it doesn't lead to addiction. A 1998 double-blind, randomized, controlled German study found valerian worked as well as the sedative benzodiazepine (*Librium*) without the withdrawal problems (Schmitz).

In the United States, valerian is used to flavor foods and soft drinks.

How It's Used

Valerian is usually taken as an herbal extract in capsules about an hour before bedtime. It also comes in a tincture, and in combination products with hops and other herbs.

Expert Opinion

This non-addicting herb might help you sleep more soundly. It's widely used in Europe as a sedative.

Cautions

! There are no known serious side effects.

! Don't drink alcohol and take valerian, or take it with other sleep aids or tranquilizers: You'll increase the sedating effects.

Vitamins and Minerals

Vitamin and mineral supplements can help with many kinds of arthritis. Although you may be eating plenty of fresh vegetables, fruit, dairy and other products high in vitamins and essential nutrients, that may not be enough. Illness, aging and the effects of prescription drugs can eat up your vitamin and mineral reserves. Often, chronic disease and medications affect your body's ability to absorb or use nutrients. And you may not be getting the proper nutrients in your diet in the first place: Pain can kill your appetite, and aching joints make it difficult to shop for healthful foods and cook.

Studies show that supplementing your diet with some vitamins and other nutrients can ease symptoms, and can help prevent other diseases connected with some kinds of arthritis such as osteoporosis and heart disease.

But that doesn't mean dosing yourself with megadoses of vitamins and minerals. Too much of a good thing can cause problems as well. It's better to eat well (see Food and Arthritis, page 159).

Here's what rheumatologists recommend and why.

Daily multivitamins. Start with a standard multivitamin, and then consider what supplements you might need to add and how much. When you consider additional supplements, see if you are already getting it in your multivitamin. If you are, be sure to add up the amount in the single supplement and the amount in the multivitamin to figure your *total* daily dosage.

Antioxidants. Antioxidants are nutrients that have been shown to destroy free radicals, the molecules that are believed to contribute to many diseases (including cancer and the arthritis conditions) and aging. Free radicals are everywhere, including in our bodies, and we need a good supply of antioxidants to keep them from doing damage.

Antioxidants include vitamins C, E and beta carotene, the trace mineral selenium and flavinoids.

Naturally occurring antioxidants such as lutein (found in leafy greens) and beta-cryptoxanthine (found in orange and yellow vegetables) have been associated with lower risks of osteoarthritis of the knee (Jordan). It's best to get these from foods, which contain the whole substances, rather than from supplements. Getting five daily servings of fruits and fresh vegetables will boost your antioxidant levels.

Vitamin A (beta carotene). Beta carotene is an anitoxidant that can protect cells. Along with vitamin E, beta carotene has been connected with a reduced risk of osteoarthritis progression (McAlindon 2). However, one study of osteoarthritis in Caucasians and African Americans found high blood levels of beta carotene were associated with an

Vitamins and Minerals

increased risk of having knee osteoarthritis (Jordan). Researchers can't explain the different results yet: It could be from different study designs or that those with higher levels of beta carotene were taking more because they had osteoarthritis.

Because of these and other studies, many nutritionists do not recommend beta carotene supplements. Talk to your doctor. If you supplement with beta carotene, the usual dosage is 2,500 IU for women, 5,000 IU for men per day. Women who are pregnant must not use beta carotene supplements as it can cause birth defects.

The B Vitamins. Several of the B vitamins are helpful for those with arthritis. You may find all of these in one B complex vitamin, or in your daily multivitamin.

Vitamin B3 (niacinamide). A National Institutes of Health study of the effect of vitamin B3 on osteoarthritis found it didn't reduce pain on its own, but that those taking NSAIDs could lower those doses by 13 percent. It also improved joint mobility compared to those taking a placebo (Jonas).

A usual dosage is 10–25 mg per day.

Vitamin B5 (panothentic acid). Some research suggests this supplement might help morning stiffness and pain from rheumatoid arthritis.

A usual dosage is 250 mg per day. However, some people with rheumatoid arthritis take 2 grams (2,000 mg) per day.

Vitamin B6. Lupus brings a special risk of heart disease, and new research shows that folic acid and B6 decrease blood levels of homocysteine, an amino acid associated with stroke and heart disease (Petri).

The usual dose is 1 mg of folic acid, and 50 mg of B6 per day.

Vitamin B12. If your diet is low in animal foods, including dairy and fish, you might need some extra B12.

A multivitamin with B12 should be enough.

Vitamin C. Examination of patients from the Framingham study (a long-term look at the health of residents of a town in Massachusetts) found that a high intake of vitamin C was associated with a three-fold decrease in the risk of osteoarthritis progression and pain.

The usual dosage is 500–1,000 mg per day. Some people take much more, but large amounts can upset your stomach or give you diarrhea. Also, if you have a hereditary disorder of iron metabolism called hemochromatosis, vitamin C supplements can increase absorption of iron, worsening the condition.

Vitamins and Minerals

Calcium. Along with Vitamin D, calcium can help protect bones and joints, prevent osteoporosis, and offset the bone-stealing effects of glucocorticoid medications such as prednisone. It's also essential to healthy skin, teeth, blood clotting and muscle contractions (muscle cramps can be due to lack of calcium). You can find calcium in dairy products and other food sources such as sardines, canned salmon, green leafy vegetables and soy products like tofu. But most people with arthritis or related diseases – and women past menopause – should be taking calcium supplements.

The usual dosage is 1,000–1,200 mg of calcium carbonate per day. Don't take calcium from oyster shells or dolomite, as these might be contaminated with heavy metals.

Men should not routinely take supplemental calcium due to the risk of renal stones.

Vitamin D. Another study based on the Framingham group found that osteoarthritis progression was three times higher in people who consumed low amounts of vitamin D (McAlindon 1). Supplemental vitamin D is found in dairy products – even those with reduced fat content. Also, vitamin D is synthesized in the body and particularly in the skin in response to sunlight. Often, elderly people in northern climates will not go outside in winter and may also avoid dairy products due to lactose intolerance.

The usual dosage is 400–800 IU per day of vitamin D.

Vitamin E. Vitamin E supplements can help reduce your risk of heart disease, and may relieve osteoarthritis symptoms. Two studies showed it eased pain better than a placebo (Machtey, Blankenhorn) and in another study it was better than an NSAID (Scherak) for pain relief. However, it may not help if you are an African American man. A study of African American men showed vitamin E had no effect on osteoarthritis of the knee (Jordan).

The usual dosage is 400–600 IU per day.

Folic acid. Many people have low levels of folic acid, which is needed for cells to reproduce. It's also needed by the body to make SAM (S-adenosylmethionine), a nutrient that protects and maintains healthy cartilage (see SAM, page 224).

Adequate folic acid levels are especially important for people with rheumatoid arthritis who are taking methotrexate. This drug reduces folic acid levels, which can lead to nausea and diarrhea. It's also recommend for those with lupus, who should take it with vitamin B6 to lower homocysteine, an amino acid associated with stroke and heart disease.

The usual dosage is 1 mg per day. Ask your doctor about the best way to take folic acid and methotrexate.

WILD YAM *(Dioscorea villosa)*

You may have been told wild yam supplements are a "natural" source of DHEA, which shows promise for treating lupus (see DHEA). That's not strictly true. Wild yam does indeed contain a "natural" source of steroids – but not in any form your body can use. The raw ingredients have to be chemically converted in a laboratory to estrogens, progesterones or other hormones before your body can access them.

Some herb guides say yams contain chemicals that could be anti-inflammatory, but there are no studies that prove this.

Expert Opinion

Don't waste your money on wild yam supplements for lupus or rheumatoid arthritis.

ZINC SULFATE

Zinc is essential to many body functions, and gained fame recently as a cold preventive. Levels are often low in those with rheumatoid arthritis, and studies have shown supplements may ease symptoms. In a small, double-blind study of people with rheumatoid arthritis, zinc sulfate improved joint swelling, morning stiffness, walking time, and the patient's own impression of overall disease activity (Simkin). Another study of patients with psoriatic arthritis who took zinc sulfate showed similar results as well as a decrease in biochemical signs of disease (Clemmensen).

How It's Used

Check with your doctor for proper dosages. See Cautions below.

Expert Opinion

Zinc supplements might help – but you may be getting enough already.

Cautions

! Zinc appears safe when taken in doses less than 50 mg per day, but doses higher than 150 mg per day can lower HDLs, the "good" cholesterol, and have other effects.

Potential Supplement-Drug Interactions

Herbs and other supplements can be powerful medicine: They can interact with each other, and with prescription or over-the-counter drugs you may be taking. Be sure you are aware of all the possible effects before you take supplements. Here are some common interactions.

BROMELAIN	May increase effects of blood-thinning drugs and tetracycline antibiotics.
CHONDROITIN	May increase effects of blood-thinning drugs and herbs.
ECHINACEA	Might counteract immune-suppressant drugs such as glucocorticoids taken for lupus and rheumatoid arthritis. Might increase side effects of methotrexate.
EVENING PRIMROSE OIL	Can counteract the effects of anti-convulsant drugs.
FISH OIL	May increase effects of blood-thinning drugs and herbs.
FOLIC ACID	Interferes with methotrexate; ask your doctor how to take it.
G.L.A.	May increase effects of blood-thinning drugs and herbs.
GARLIC	Can increase effects of blood-thinning drugs and herbs.
GINGER	Can increase NSAID side effects and effects of blood-thinning drugs and herbs.
GINKGO	May increase effects of blood-thinning drugs and herbs.
GINSENG	May increase effects of blood-thinning drugs, estrogens and glucocorticoids; shouldn't be used by those with diabetes; may interact with MAO inhibitors.
KAVA KAVA	Can increase effects of alcohol, sedatives and tranquilizers.
MAGNESIUM	May interact with blood pressure medications.
ST. JOHN'S WORT	May enhance effects of narcotics, alcohol, and antidepressants; increase risk of sunburn; interfere with iron absorption.
VALERIAN	Can increase the effects of sedatives and tranquilizers.
ZINC	Can interfere with glucocorticoids and other immunosuppressing drugs.

Those in the studies took high doses – so check with your doctor about the right dosage for you.

! It's often combined with other trace minerals or added to multiple vitamins, so check the labels to see how much you may already be getting before you supplement.

! It can work against glucocorticoids and other immunosuppressing drugs, so check with your doctor if you are taking these.

IS IT ARTHRITIS?

Chances are you or someone you know has a form of arthritis or a related condition. These conditions cause pain, stiffness and sometimes swelling in or around joints. This can make it difficult to do the movements you rely on every day for working or taking care of your family. But you can take steps now to avoid arthritis or to reduce pain and keep moving.

Arthritis affects one in every seven Americans. It affects people of all ages, but it occurs more often as a person gets older. Some forms, however, often begin between ages 20 and 40. Arthritis is usually chronic, meaning that it lasts a long time; for many people, it may not go away.

If you have any of these signs in or around a joint for more than two weeks, it's time to see your doctor. These symptoms can develop suddenly or slowly. Only a doctor can tell if it's arthritis.

Warning Signs

Pain from arthritis can be ongoing or can come and go. It may occur when you're moving or after you have been still for some time. You may feel pain in one spot or in many parts of your body.

Warning Signs of Arthritis
- Pain
- Stiffness
- Swelling (sometimes)
- Difficulty moving a joint

Your joints may feel stiff and be hard to move. You may find that it's hard to do daily tasks you used to do easily, such as climbing stairs or opening a jar. Pain and stiffness usually will be more severe in the morning or after periods of inactivity.

In some types of inflammatory arthritis, the skin over the joint may appear swollen and red, and feel warm to the touch. Some types of arthritis can also be associated with fatigue.

Causes

There are more than 100 different types of arthritis and related conditions. The cause of most types is unknown. Because there are so many different types, there are likely to be many different causes.

Scientists are currently studying what roles three major factors play in certain types of arthritis. These include the genetic factors you inherit from your parents, events during your life, and other lifestyle factors. The importance of these lifestyle and environmental factors varies for every type of arthritis.

CAN YOU PREVENT IT?

There are steps you can take to reduce your risk for getting certain types of arthritis or to reduce disability if you already have arthritis. These steps for preventing arthritis are discussed in the following sections.

If You Don't Have Arthritis

It's important to maintain your recommended weight, especially as you get older. People who are overweight have a higher frequency of osteoarthritis. Excess weight increases your risk for developing osteoarthritis in the knees, and possibly in the hips and hands. Women are especially at risk for this. In men, excess weight increases the risk for developing gout.

What if you're already overweight? Research shows that middle-age and older women of average height who lose 11 pounds or more over 10 years cut their risk for developing knee osteoarthritis in half. To lose weight, try exercising and eating fewer calories. If you're having trouble with weight control, ask your doctor or a registered dietitian for help.

Joint injuries caused by accidents, injuries or overuse increase your risk for osteoarthritis. Keeping the muscles around joints strong – especially the knee – may reduce the risk of wear on that joint and help prevent injury. You can also inherit certain genes that may increase your risk for some types of arthritis. More research is needed to find out how to reduce your risk from these factors.

If You Have Arthritis

What can you do to maintain your independence if you already have arthritis? Studies show that exercise helps reduce the pain and fatigue of many different kinds of arthritis and related diseases. Exercise keeps you moving, working and doing daily activities that help you remain independent. Read the exercise section on page 245 of this appendix for tips to help you start or maintain an exercise program.

It's also important to control your weight if you have knee or back osteoarthritis. Being overweight puts you at risk for more severe disease, and for getting osteoarthritis in your other knee if only one is affected now.

HOW IS ARTHRITIS DIAGNOSED?

It's important to find out if you have arthritis and what type it is because treatments vary for each type. Early diagnosis and treatment are important to help slow or prevent damage to joints that can occur during the first few years for several types.

Only a doctor can determine if you have arthritis and what type it is. When you see your doctor for the first time about arthritis, expect at least three things to happen. Your doctor will ask questions about your symptoms, examine you, and possibly order some tests or X-rays.

You can help your doctor by writing down the answers to the following considerations before your appointment. Bring your answers when you see your doctor.

What to Tell Your Doctor

- Where it hurts
- When it hurts
- When it first began to hurt
- How long it has hurt
- If you have seen any swelling
- What daily tasks are hard to do now
- If you have ever hurt the joint in an accident or overused it on the job or in a hobby
- If anyone in your family has had similar problems

Arthritis may limit how far or how easily you can move a joint. Your doctor may move the joint that hurts or ask you to move it. This is to see how far the joint moves or if it moves through its normal range of motion. Your doctor will also check for swelling, tender points, skin rashes or problems with other parts of your body.

Finally, your doctor may conduct some tests. These may include tests of your blood, urine or joint fluid. They also may include X-rays of your joints. The tests help confirm what type of arthritis your doctor suspects based on your medical history and physical exam and help rule out other diseases that cause similar symptoms.

What Your Doctor Should Tell You

- If it's arthritis or a related condition
- What type it is
- What to expect
- What you can do about it

The results from your medical history, physical exam and tests help your doctor match your symptoms to the pattern for a specific disease. It may take several visits before your doctor can tell what type of arthritis you have. Symptoms for some types of arthritis develop slowly and may appear similar to other types in early stages. Your doctor may suspect a certain type of arthritis, but may watch how your symptoms develop over time to confirm it.

What type of doctor should you see for arthritis? Your family doctor may be able to diagnose and treat common types of arthritis if he or she is up-to-date on arthritis diagnosis and treatments. However, your doctor may need to refer you to an arthritis specialist for the diagnosis or for special care. Arthritis specialists are called rheumatologists. You can ask your local Arthritis Foundation for a list of arthritis specialists in your area.

WHAT'S YOUR TYPE?

There are more than 100 different types of arthritis and related diseases. It is important to know which type of arthritis you have so you can treat it properly. If you don't know which type you have, call your doctor or ask during your next visit.

Arthritis most often affects areas in or around joints, which are parts of the body where bones meet, such as your knee. The ends of the bones are covered by cartilage, a spongy material that acts as a shock absorber to keep bones from rubbing together. The joint is enclosed in a capsule and lined with tissue called the synovium. The synovium produces a slippery fluid that helps the joint move smoothly and easily. Muscles and tendons support the joint and help you move.

Different types of arthritis can affect one or more parts of a joint. This may result in a change of shape and alignment in the joints.

Certain types of arthritis can also affect other parts of the body such as the skin and internal organs.

Overviews of some common types of arthritis and related conditions are described on the following pages.

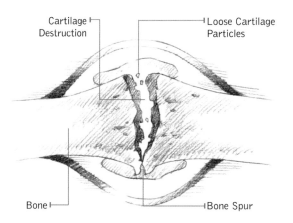

Joint with osteoarthritis

Osteoarthritis

The most common type of arthritis is osteoarthritis, or OA. It affects many of us as we grow older. It is sometimes called degenerative arthritis because it involves the breakdown of cartilage and bones, causing pain and stiffness. Osteoarthritis usually affects the fingers and weight-bearing joints, including the knees, feet, hips and back. It affects both

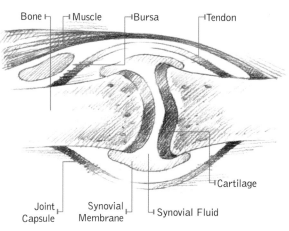

Different types of arthritis can affect different parts of a joint.

Appendix A: Arthritis Answers

men and women and usually occurs after age
45. Treatments for OA include pain relievers
or anti-inflammatory drugs, exercise, heat or
cold, joint protection, pacing your activities,
self-care skills, and sometimes surgery.

Rheumatoid Arthritis

In rheumatoid arthritis (RA), an abnor-
mality in the body's defense or immune system causes inflammation of the joints.
Inflammation begins in the joint lining and
then may damage both cartilage and bone.
Rheumatoid arthritis often affects the same
joints on both sides of the body. The hands,
wrists, feet, knees, ankles, shoulders, neck,
jaw and elbows can be affected. Rheumatoid
arthritis is more common in women than in
men. Conventional treatments include disease-modifying and anti-inflammatory
drugs, exercise, heat or cold, rest, joint protection, self-care skills, and sometimes
surgery.

Fibromyalgia

Fibromyalgia is a condition that affects
muscles and their attachments to bone. It is
characterized by widespread pain and tender
points, which are certain places on the body
that are more sensitive to pain. People with
fibromyalgia frequently experience fatigue,
disturbed sleep, stiffness and sometimes psychological distress. Fibromyalgia is a common

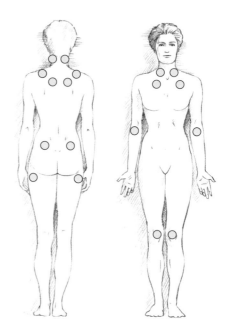

Some of the tender points that are
common in fibromyalgia.

condition, and it usually affects women.
Treatments include exercise, sleep improvement, pacing your activities, self-care
skills and medication, as well as complementary therapies.

Osteoporosis

Osteoporosis is a disease that causes bone
to lose mass and become brittle, often leading
to painful fractures and/or rounded shoulders
and loss of height. The disease affects more
than 25 million Americans, 80 percent of
whom are women. It is the major underlying
cause of bone fractures in postmenopausal

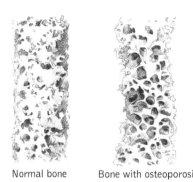

Normal bone   Bone with osteoporosis

Osteoporosis makes bone less dense and more susceptible to fractures.

common symptoms include a butterfly-shaped rash over the cheeks and across the bridge of the nose; scaly, disc-shaped sores on the face, neck and/or chest; abnormal sun sensitivity; and arthritis.) Lupus occurs more often in African Americans than in Caucasians, and may also occur more frequently in Asian and Latino populations. Lupus is treatable, but can be quite serious. Conventional treatments include taking medications to reduce inflammation or reduce the immune system's activity, balancing rest with exercise, and eating a proper diet.

women and the elderly. People with some forms of arthritis (such as RA) are also at risk for developing osteoporosis because certain medications (such as glucocorticoids) can cause loss of bone mass and contribute to osteoporosis. Many of the steps you can take to prevent osteoporosis – increasing calcium and vitamin D intake, taking medications to reduce bone loss, exercising regularly, and maintaining a healthy lifestyle – also can help treat it. Your doctor can help determine which treatments are best for you.

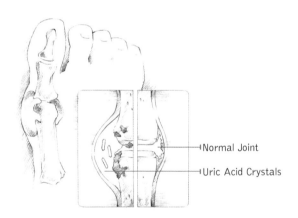

Normal Joint

Uric Acid Crystals

Joint with gout compared with a normal joint

Lupus

Lupus is a rheumatic disease that affects the skin and body tissues, and possibly organs such as the kidneys, lungs or heart. Lupus affects women about eight to 10 times more often than men. Symptoms often first appear in women between ages 18 and 45. (A few

Gout

Gout results when the body produces too much or is unable to rid itself of a natural substance called uric acid. The uric acid forms needlelike crystals in the joint that cause severe pain and swelling. Gout usually affects the big toes, ankles and knees. More men than women have gout. Conventional treatments include anti-inflammatory and special gout drugs, weight reduction and limiting alcohol intake.

Low Back Pain

Low back pain can result from a back strain or injury or from certain types of arthritis. Treatments include pain relievers or anti-inflammatory drugs, exercise, heat or cold, joint protection, pacing your activities, and self-care skills.

Bursitis and Tendinitis

Bursitis and tendinitis result from irritation caused by injuring or overusing a joint. Bursitis affects a small sac that helps muscles move easily; tendinitis affects the tendons that attach muscle to bone. (See the illustration of a normal joint on page 239 to see where tendons and bursae are located.) Treatments include anti-inflammatory drugs, heat or cold, and rest.

There are many more types of arthritis and related conditions, including ankylosing spondylitis, juvenile rheumatoid arthritis, polymyalgia rheumatica and psoriatic arthritis. The Arthritis Foundation has educational brochures about these and many more types.

WHO MAY HELP TREAT YOU?

Part of your conventional treatment plan may involve working with different health-care specialists such as those listed below.

Family physicians and general practitioners provide medical care for adults and for children with different types of arthritis. These doctors also can help you find a specialist, if necessary.

Internists specialize in internal medicine and in the treatment of adult diseases. They provide general care to adults and often help select specialists. Internists should not be confused with interns, who are doctors doing a year's training in a hospital after medical school.

Rheumatologists specialize in treating people with arthritis or related diseases that affect the joints, muscles, bones, skin and other tissues. You may see a rheumatologist for diagnosis and for appropriate, up-to-date treatment of your condition. Most rheumatologists are internists who have had further training in the care of people with arthritis and related conditions. Some rheumatologists also have training in pediatrics.

Ophthalmic specialists provide eye care and treatment.

Orthopaedic surgeons may be consulted to perform certain surgical procedures if your joints are damaged.

Pediatricians treat childhood diseases.

Physiatrists may direct your physical therapy and rehabilitation activities.

Podiatrists are experts in foot care. If arthritis affects your feet, a podiatrist can prescribe special supports and shoes.

Psychiatrists are physicians who treat mental or emotional problems that may need special attention.

Nurses trained in arthritis care assist your doctor with your treatment. They also help teach you about your treatment program and can answer many of your questions.

Occupational therapists can teach you how to reduce strain on your joints while doing everyday activities. They can fit you with splints and other devices to help reduce stress on your joints.

Pharmacists fill your prescriptions for medicines and can explain the drugs' actions and side effects. Pharmacists can tell you how different medicines work together, and they can also answer questions about over-the-counter medicines.

Physical therapists can show you exercises to help keep your muscles strong and your joints from becoming stiff. They can help you learn how to use special equipment to move better. Some physical therapists also are trained to design individualized fitness programs for cardiovascular health maintenance and weight control.

Psychologists can help you with emotional or mental problems.

Social workers can help you find solutions to social and financial problems related to your disease.

WHAT TREATMENTS WORK?

Before beginning your treatment, your doctor should diagnose which type of arthritis or related condition you have. Once this is determined, there are many things that help reduce pain, relieve stiffness and keep you moving. Your care may involve more than one kind of treatment. Your doctor may recommend medications, but there are many things you can do on your own to help manage pain and fatigue and move easier.

Finding the right treatment takes time, and can involve trial and error until you and your doctor find what works best. Be sure to let your doctor know if a treatment is not working. Your treatment may also change as your arthritis changes.

Conventional treatments for arthritis can be divided into several categories described on the following pages. You can take steps in each of these areas to help yourself feel better and move easier.

Medication

Many different drugs are used to treat arthritis and related diseases; the ones your doctor prescribes will depend on the type of arthritis you have. Some medications are available without a prescription, but others must be prescribed by your doctor. You should always check with your doctor before taking any medication, even over-the-counter drugs. Your doctor can tell you how much and when to take them for best relief, as well as how to avoid any drug-related problems.

Aspirin-free pain relievers (analgesics) may be recommended by your doctor if you just need pain relief, are allergic to aspirin, or have had an ulcer. Acetaminophen gives temporary relief of noninflammatory or mild arthritis pain, but does not reduce swelling. It is available without a prescription.

Anti-inflammatory drugs reduce both pain and swelling. These medications are called nonsteroidal anti-inflammatory drugs (NSAIDs). Some NSAIDs such as aspirin, ibuprofen and naproxen are available at a lower dose without a prescription; others are only available by prescription. The most common side effect of these drugs is stomach upset. Stop the medication and call your doctor if stomach pain from taking NSAIDs is more than mild and if it persists.

Know About Your Medications

Make sure to find out the following information about your medications from your doctor:

- Its name
- How much to take
- How and when to take it
- How quickly it works
- What benefits to expect
- When to contact your doctor if you don't get relief
- Side effects to watch for
- Other drugs to avoid taking with it

Biologic agents affect the immune system cells involved in rheumatoid arthritis to help reduce pain and inflammation. These drugs are used in patients who have not found adequate relief from other treatments.

Glucocorticoids are prescribed to reduce severe pain and inflammation. They are given by injection or in pill form. Injections can bring quick relief, but can only be used several times in one year because they may weaken bone, tendons and cartilage. Because of potentially serious side effects, glucocorticoids must be prescribed and monitored by a doctor.

Disease modifiers (DMARDs) tend to slow down the disease process in rheumatoid arthritis and other types of inflammatory arthritis. These medications include sulfasalazine, methotrexate and antibiotics, as well as more experimental drugs. They are available only by prescription and may take several weeks or months to work. Your doctor will carefully monitor you for side effects from taking these powerful drugs.

Sleep medications may promote deeper sleep and help relax muscles. These drugs may help people with fibromyalgia sleep better. They are available by prescription and are used in very low doses at bedtime.

Exercise

Regular exercise is important to keep you moving and independent. Exercise helps lessen pain, increase movement, reduce fatigue, and helps you look and feel better. Three types of exercises can help people with arthritis.

Range-of-motion exercises reduce stiffness. They keep your joints flexible by moving them to their fullest extent. Do these exercises daily.

Strengthening exercises increase or maintain muscle strength. Strong muscles help keep your joints stable and make it easier to move. Do these exercises daily or every other day.

Endurance exercises build fitness. They help keep your heart healthy and control your weight. You should exercise for a total of 20 to 30 minutes, three times a week, at a pace that raises or sustains your heart rate. You can build your endurance by exercising for shorter periods several times a day.

Plan your exercises at times of the day when you have less stiffness or pain. Start slowly. Build up the amount of time you exercise and the number of repetitions you do. Exercise at a level that allows you to talk comfortably during the activity. If pain from exercise lasts more than two hours, you may have done too much. Reduce your level of activity next time. Stop exercising right away if you have chest pains, severe dizziness or shortness of breath, or if you feel sick to your stomach.

The Arthritis Foundation offers several water and land exercise classes and videos. Call your local Arthritis Foundation office to learn more about the classes or to order exercise videos. You can also read the Arthritis Foundation's booklet *Exercise and Your Arthritis* for information on exercising safely.

Heat and Cold

Using heat or cold over joints or muscles may give you short-term relief from pain and stiffness. You can also use heat or cold to help prepare for exercise. Some people feel better using heat; others prefer cold.

Heat helps relax aching muscles. Sources of heat include hot packs, hot tubs or heated pools. Cold numbs the area so you don't feel as much pain. You can apply cold with ice, cold packs or even bags of frozen vegetables.

It's important to use heat and cold safely. Do not use either treatment for more than 20 minutes at a time. Let your skin return to normal temperature between applications. Don't use heat with rubs or creams because this can result in skin burns.

For more information on using heat and cold correctly, talk to your physical therapist. You can also read the Arthritis Foundation booklet *Managing Your Pain* for more tips.

Pacing Activities

Pacing yourself saves energy by switching periods of activity with periods of rest. Pacing helps protect your joints from the stress of repeated tasks, and helps reduce fatigue.

Alternate heavy or repeated tasks with easy ones. Change tasks often so you don't hold joints in one position for a long time. Plan rest breaks during your daily activities.

Joint Protection

You can protect your joints by using them in ways that avoid excess stress. Protecting your joints makes it easier to do daily tasks. There are three methods of joint protection.

Paying attention to joint position means using joints in the best way to avoid excess stress on them. Use larger or stronger joints to carry things. For instance, carry your grocery bags using your forearms or palms instead of your fingers.

Using walking or assistive devices can help keep stress off certain joints. Your doctor may suggest using a cane, crutches or a walker to reduce stress on your hips and knees.

Many assistive devices have special features that help make tasks easier. Special features, such as extra thick pens, make them easier to hold and write. Longer handles and reachers give you better leverage. Lightweight items, such as plastic dishes, are easier to carry.

You can read the Arthritis Foundation booklet *Managing Your Activities* for tips on protecting your joints and using them wisely.

Weight control involves staying close to your recommended weight, or losing weight if you are overweight now. This has a number of benefits. Weight control helps reduce your risk for developing osteoarthritis in the knees or gout. If you already have knee osteoarthritis, losing weight may lessen pain by reducing stress on your joints. Exercising and reducing calories will help you lose weight. If you need to lose a lot of weight, work with your doctor and a registered or licensed dietitian to find the best weight-loss program for you.

Surgery

Most people with arthritis will never need surgery. However, surgery can help in some cases when other treatments have failed. It can reduce pain and increase movement.

Two kinds of surgery help people with arthritis. Synovectomy repairs the existing joint by removing debris, and fusing or correcting bone deformity. Joint replacement surgery replaces the damaged joint with an artificial one.

Orthopaedic surgeons are the doctors who perform most joint replacements. Plastic surgeons may help with hand surgery. If your doctor suggests surgery, you may want to ask another doctor for a second opinion.

Self-Care Skills

Arthritis and related conditions may affect you in different ways, from what you can do to how you look. Daily tasks may be harder to do or may take longer. Arthritis may change the shape of your joints, but most people won't be able to tell by looking at you that you have arthritis.

You are the best manager for your arthritis. Being a good arthritis manager means understanding your disease and knowing what to expect. It also means planning your activities for your best times or days and learning how to work with your doctor as a team. This includes discussing changes in your abilities, what works and what doesn't.

You can help yourself feel better by learning to manage your symptoms and how they affect your daily activities. You can also learn skills to help manage how arthritis affects your emotions and your family.

Symptom-management skills use problem-solving methods to help you identify and overcome difficulties with daily tasks. You can learn skills to help you exercise and use heat or cold. You can protect your joints and pace your daily schedule to reduce fatigue and stress on the joints. You can learn all these skills through an Arthritis Foundation Self-Help Course or video.

Coping skills can help you manage the changes arthritis and other diseases can bring to your life. Pain, stress, and changes in roles and your physical appearance can cause depression. Use mental exercises and things you enjoy doing to relieve stress. Talk about the changes arthritis brings and share your feelings with family and friends. Ask for help when you need it. You can find understanding from others coping with arthritis in an Arthritis Foundation support group.

WHAT'S NEW IN ARTHRITIS RESEARCH?

Progress is so fast in some areas of arthritis research today that the media often report new findings before the medical journal with the information reaches your doctor's office. As a result, you need to know how to evaluate reports on new arthritis research.

Arthritis researchers are looking at four broad areas of research. These include causes, treatments, education and lifestyle influences.

In osteoarthritis, researchers are looking for ways to stop the destruction of cartilage and ways to rebuild it. For rheumatoid arthritis and other conditions that involve inflammation, researchers are trying to understand the steps that lead to inflammation and how it can be slowed or stopped.

What to Look for in News About Arthritis Research

When you read about a new finding in arthritis research, ask these questions:

- Is this research associated with a medical facility?
- Is there a scientific reason to think the results are reliable?
- Were the people in the study like you — the same age, sex and type of arthritis?
- Has the research been published in a medical journal?
- Does the report suggest health actions that people with your type of arthritis should take as a result of the research?

Your doctor can tell you about other new research findings. If you would like to take part in arthritis research, ask your doctor for a referral to a study in your area.

Many people help make arthritis research possible. The federal government, through its National Institutes of Health, is the largest supporter of arthritis research. Drug companies conduct research on new medications.

The Arthritis Foundation is the largest private, nonprofit source of funds for arthritis research. Your contributions help the Arthritis Foundation support grants to train young scientists or fund studies by more experienced researchers. In addition, the Arthritis Foundation advocates strongly for increased government-sponsored arthritis research.

FOR MORE INFORMATION

Contact your local Arthritis Foundation office for a list of free brochures about different forms of arthritis and related conditions, treatment options, and self-management techniques. The following services may also be available in your area:

- **Self-help courses** – Learn how to take control of your own care in these courses designed for people with arthritis, lupus and fibromyalgia.
- **Warm-water exercise program** – Join in the fun of a six- to 10-week exercise program in a heated pool.

- **Land exercise programs** – Move easier in several levels of exercise classes, or exercise at home by purchasing an Arthritis Foundation exercise videotape.
- **Support groups and clubs** – Share your successes and problems with others, and get tips on how to overcome challenges caused by arthritis.

THE ARTHRITIS FOUNDATION

The Arthritis Foundation is the source of help and hope for the nearly 43 million Americans who have arthritis, rheumatic diseases or related musculoskeletal conditions. The Foundation supports research to cure and prevent arthritis and seeks to improve the quality of life for those affected by arthritis.

Formed in 1948, the Foundation is the only national, voluntary health organization that works for all people affected by any of the more than 100 forms of arthritis or related diseases. Volunteers in chapters nationwide help to support research, professional and community education programs, services for people with arthritis, government advocacy and fund-raising activities.

The American Juvenile Arthritis Organization (AJAO) is composed of children, parents, health professionals, teachers and others concerned specifically about juvenile arthritis. A council of the Arthritis Foundation, AJAO focuses its efforts on the specific problems related to arthritis in children.

As a not-for-profit organization, the Arthritis Foundation relies on your contributions to fund research, programs and services. You can make a difference in people's lives by becoming a member of the Arthritis Foundation. Please contact your local chapter to receive materials about the benefits of membership, including the award-winning bimonthly magazine *Arthritis Today*.

Here are some books and Web sites about alternative medicine that are trustworthy and of interest. Look also at the Resources at the end of each therapy type for books, Web sites and other resources about that therapy.

BOOKS

Afterwards, You're a Genius: Faith, Medicine, and the Metaphysics of Healing, by Chip Brown. 1998. Penguin. Hardcover. $24.95.

Alternative Medicine: What Works, by Adriane Fugh-Berman. 1997. Baltimore, MD: Williams & Wilkins. Paperback. $14.95.

American Holistic Health Association Complete Guide to Alternative Medicine, by William Collinge, MPH, PhD. 1996. Warner Books. Hardcover. $24.95.

8 Weeks to Optimum Health: A Proven Program for Taking Full Advantage of Your Body's Natural Healing Power, by Andrew Weil, MD. 1998. Fawcett Books. Paperback. $13.95.

Health and Healing: Understanding Conventional and Alternative Medicine, by Andrew Weil, MD. 1998. Boston: Houghton Mifflin. Chapters Publications. Paperback. $13.

The Healthy Mind Healthy Body Handbook, by David S. Sobel, MD and Robert Ornstein, PhD. 1997. Los Altos, CA: ISHK Book Service. Paperback. $15.

Living a Healthy Life with Chronic Illness, by Kate Lorig, Halstead Holman, Diana Lauren, Virginia Gonzalez, Marian Minor. 1994. Palo Alto, CA: Bull Publications. Paperback. $16.95.

Love, Medicine and Miracles: Lessons Learned About Self-Healing from a Surgeon's Experience With Exceptional Patients, by Bernic S. Siegel. 1990. Harper Perennial Library. Paperback. $14.

Manifesto for a New Medicine: Your Guide to Healing Partnerships and the Wise Use of Alternative Therapies, by James S. Gordon. 1997. Perseus. Paperback. $13.

Nature's Cures, by Michael Castleman. 1996. Emmaus, PA. Rodale Press, Inc. Hardcover. $27.95.

When Things Fall Apart: Heart Advice for Difficult Times, by Pema Chodron. 1997. Shambhala Publications. Paperback. $20. Also available on audio tape.

WEB SITES

Be aware that online addresses and contents change frequently. Listing these sites does not imply approval of the content by the Arthritis Foundation.

Altmednet.com
Web site: http://www.altmednet.com
Sponsored by American Health Consultants, a producer of health-care information, this site is aimed at medical professionals. It has many alternative medicine links.

Arthritis Foundation
Web site: http://www.arthritis.org

Ask Dr. Weil
Web site: http://www.drwcil.com
The Web site of Andrew Weil, MD, has a list of practitioners and links to useful information.

Ask NOAH
Web site: http://www.noah.cuny.edu
Excellent information about many health issues, including alternative practices, is available on The New York Online Access to Health (NOAH). It's in English and Spanish.

Health World Online
Web site: http://www.healthy.net
An online resources center for health information, including alternative therapies.

National Center for Complementary and Alternative Medicine
Web site: http://nccam.nih.gov
This arm of the National Institutes of Health conducts and supports research and supplies information on complementary and alternative medicine.

National Council Against Health Fraud
Web site: http://ncahf.org
A critical – and sometimes negative – look at unconventional therapies.

The Rosenthal Center for Complementary and Alternative Medicine
Web site: http://cpmcnet.columbia.edu/dept/rosenthal
This site is posted by the Columbia University College of Physicians and Surgeons. It contains a database directory, fact sheets on complementary therapies and training, and other information.

University of Maryland Complementary Medicine Program
Web site: http://www.compmed.ummc.ab.umd.edu
Contains information on research in complementary therapies and pain conditions. Also has a database of scientific literature in complementary medicine and pain.

World Health Organization
Web site: http://www.who.org

ALTERNATIVE HEALING SYSTEMS

Andrade LE, Ferraz MD, Atra E, Castro A, Silva MS. A randomized controlled trial to evaluate the effectiveness of homeopathy in rheumatoid arthritis. *Scand J Rheumatol* 1999 20(3):203-8

Bensoussan A, Talley NJ, Hing M, Menzies R, Guo A, Ngu M. Treatment of irritable bowel syndrome with Chinese herbal medicine: a randomized controlled trial. *JAMA* 1998;280:1585-9

Berkson DL. Osteoarthritis, chiropractic, and nutrition: osteoarthritis considered as a natural part of a three stage subluxation complex: its reversibility: its relevance and treatability by chiropractic and nutritional correlates. *Med Hypotheses* 1991 Dec;36(4):356-67

Blunt KL, Rajwani MH, Guerriero RC. The effectiveness of chiropractic management of fibromyalgia patients: a pilot study. *J Manipulative Physiol Ther* 1997 Jul-Aug;20(6):389-99
Comment in: *J Manipulative Physiol Ther* 1998 May;21(4):307
Comment in: *J Manipulative Physiol Ther 1998* Jul-Aug;21(6):429

Cherkin DC, Deyo RA, Battie M, Street J, Barlow W. A comparison of physical therapy, chiropractic manipulation, and provision of an educational booklet for the treatment of patients with low back pain. *N Engl J Med* 1998 Oct 8;339(15):1021-9

Fisher P, Greenwood A, Huskisson, Turner P, Belon P. Effect of homeopathic treatment on fibrosis. *Br Med J* 1989; 299:365-66

Gibson RG, Gibson SL, MacNeill AD, Buchanan WW. Homoeopathic therapy in rheumatoid arthritis: evaluation by double- blind clinical therapeutic trial. *Br J Clin Pharmacol* 1980 9(5):453-9

Linde K, Clausius N, Ramirez G, Melchart D, Eitel F, Hedges LV, Jonas WB. Are the clinical effects of homeopathy placebo effects? A meta-analysis of placebo-controlled trials [see comments] [published erratum appears in *Lancet* 1998 Jan 17;351(9097):220] *Lancet* 1997 Sep 20;350(9081):834-43
Comment in: *Lancet* 1997 Sep 20;350(9081):824
Comment in: *Lancet* 1997 Sep 20;350(9081):825
Comment in: *Lancet* 1998 Jan 31;351(9099):365; discussion 367-8
Comment in: *Lancet* 1998 Jan 31;351(9099):365-6; discussion 367-8
Comment in: *Lancet* 1998 Jan 31;351(9099):366; discussion 367-8
Comment in: *Lancet* 1998 Jan 31;351(9099):366-7; discussion 367-8
Comment in: *Lancet* 1998 Jan 31;351(9099):367
Comment in: *Lancet* 1998 Jan 31;351(9099):368

Shipley M, Berry H, Broster G, Jenkins M, Clover A, Williams I. Controlled trial of homoeopathic treatment of osteoarthritis. *Lancet* 1983 Jan 15;1(8316):97-8

MIND, BODY AND SPIRIT

Achterberg J, McGraw P, Lawlis GF. Rheumatoid arthritis: a study of relaxation and temperature biofeedback training as an adjunctive therapy. *Biofeedback Self Regul* 1981 Jun;6(2):207-23

Bennett RM, Burckhardt CS, Clark SR, O'Reilly CA, Wiens AN, Campbell SM. Group treatment of fibromyalgia: a 6 month outpatient program. *J Rheumatol* 1996; 23(3):521-8

Benson H; Friedman R. Harnessing the power of the placebo effect and renaming it "remembered wellness." *Annu Rev Med* 1996;47:193-9.

Blanchard EB, Greene B, Scharff L. Schwartz-McMorris SP. Relaxation training as a treatment for irritable bowel syndrome. *Biofeedback Self Regul* 1993 Sep;18(3):125-32

Bradley LA, et al. Effects of psychological therapy on pain behavior of rheumatoid arthritis patients. Treatment outcome and six-month followup. *Arthritis Rheum* 1987 Oct;30(10):1105-14

Broderick J. Mind-body medicine in rheumatological disease. *Rheum Dis Clin North Am.* 1999; Vol. 25 (suppl).

Buckelew SP, Conway R, Parker J, Deuser WE, Read J, Witty TE, Hewett JE, Minor M, Johnson JC, Van Male L, McIntosh MJ, Nigh M, Kay. Biofeedback/relaxation training and exercise interventions for fibromyalgia: a prospective trial. *Arthritis Care Res* 1998;11(3):196-209

Creamer PB, Singh B, Berman MC. Hochberg Evidence of sustained improvement from a "mind-body" intervention in patients with fibromyalgia (fm) [Abstract] Arthritis Rheum 1998; 41(suppl):S258

Domangue BB, Margolis CG, Lieberman D, Kaji H. Biochemical correlates of hypnoanalgesia in arthritic pain patients. *J Clin Psychiatry* 1985;46(6):235-8

Haanen HC, Hoenderdos HT, van Romunde LK, Hop WC, Mallee C, Terwiel JP, Hekster GB. Controlled trial of hypnotherapy in the treatment of refractory fibromyalgia. *J Rheumatol* 1991;18(1):72-5

Harvey RF, Hinton RA, Gunary RM, Barry RE. Individual and group hypnotherapy in treatment of refractory irritable bowel syndrome. *Lancet* 1989;1

Jevning R, Wilson AF, Davidson JM. Adrenocortical activity during meditation. *Hormones & Behavior* 2-1978 10(1):54-60

Kabat-Zinn J. An outpatient program in behavioral medicine for chronic pain patients based on the practice of mindfulness meditation: theoretical considerations and preliminary results. *General Hospital Psychiatry* 1982; 4(1): 33-47

Kabat-Zinn J, Lipworth L, Burney R, Sellers W. Four year follow-up of a meditation-based program for the self-regulation of chronic pain: treatment outcomes and compliance. *Clin J Pain* 1986;2:159-73

Kabat-Zinn J, Lipworth L, Burney R. The clinical use of mindfulness meditation for the self-regulation of chronic pain. *J Behav Med* 1985 Jun;8(2):163-90

Kabat-Zinn J, Wheeler E, Light T, Skillings A, Scharf MJ, Cropley TG, Hosmer D, Bernhard JD. Influence of a mindfulness meditation-based stress reduction intervention on rates of skin clearing in patients with moderate to severe psoriasis undergoing phototherapy (UVB) and photochemotherapy (PUVA). *Psychosom Med* 1998;60:625-32

Appendix C: References

Mind, Body and Spirit continued.

Kaplan KH, Goldenberg DL, Galvin-Nadeau M. The impact of a meditation-based stress reduction program on fibromyalgia. *Gen Hosp Psychiatry* 1993 Sep;15(5):284-9

Lavigne JV, Ross CK, Berry SL, Hayford JR, Pachman LM. Evaluation of a psychological treatment package for treating pain in juvenile rheumatoid arthritis. *Arthritis Care Res* 1992 Jun;5(2):101-10

Maguire BL. The effects of imagery on attitudes and moods in multiple sclerosis patients. *Altern Ther Health Med* 1996 Sep;2(5):75-9

Orme-Johnson D. Medical care utilization and the transcendental meditation program. *Psychosomatic Medicine.* 1987; 49:493-507.

Parker JC, et al. Pain management in rheumatoid arthritis patients. A cognitive-behavioral approach. *Arthritis Rheum* 1988 May;31(5):593-601

Parker JC, et al. Effects of stress management on clinical outcomes in rheumatoid arthritis. *Arthritis Rheum* 1995 Dec;38(12):1807-18

Platania-Solazzo, et al. Relaxation therapy reduces anxiety in child and adolescent psychiatric patients. *Acta Paedopsychiatrica* 1992 55(2):115-120

Shaw G; Srivastava ED; Sadlier M; Swann P; James JY; Rhodes J. Stress management for irritable bowel syndrome: a controlled trial. *Digestion* 1991;50(1):36-42

Simonton OC, Matthews-Simonton S; Sparks TF. Psychological intervention in the treatment of cancer. *Psychosomatics.* 1980;21:226-7, 231-3.

Singh BB, Berman BM, Hadhazy VA, Creamer P. A pilot study of cognitive behavioral therapy in fibromyalgia. *Altern Ther Health Med* 1998 Mar;4(2):67-70

Smyth J, Stone A, Hurewitz A, Kaell A. Effects of writing about stressful experiences on symptom reduction in patients with asthma or rheumatoid arthritis: a randomized trial. *JAMA.* 1999;281:1304-1309.

Spiegel D, Moore R. Imagery and hypnosis in the treatment of cancer patients. *Oncology* 1997 Aug;11(8):1179-89; discussion 1189-95

Spiegel D, Bloom JR. Group therapy and hypnosis reduce metastatic breast carcinoma pain. *Psychosom Med* 1983 Aug;45(4):333-9

Superio-Cabuslay, E, Ward MM, Lorig KR. Patient education interventions in osteoarthritis and rheumatoid arthritis: a meta-analytic comparison with nonsteroidal antiinflammatory drug treatment. *Arthritis Care Res* 1996 Aug;9(4):292-301

Walco GA, Varni JW, Ilowite NT. Cognitive-behavioral pain management in children with juvenile rheumatoid arthritis. *Pediatrics* 1992 Jun;89(6 Pt 1):1075-9

Walco GA, Ilowite NT. Cognitive-behavioral intervention for juvenile primary fibromyalgia syndrome. *J Rheumatol* 1992;19:1617-9

Wallace KG. Analysis of recent literature concerning relaxation and imagery interventions for cancer pain. *Cancer Nurs* 1997 Apr;20(2):79-87

Whorwell PJ, Prior A, Colgan SM. Hypnotherapy in severe irritable bowel syndrome: further experience. *Gut* 1987;28:423-5

Yocum DE, Hodes R, Sundstrom WR, Cleeland CS. Use of biofeedback training in treatment of Raynaud's disease and phenomenon. *J Rheumatol* 1985 Feb;12(1):90-3

Young LD, Bradley LA, Turner RA. Decreases in health care resource utilization in patients with rheumatoid arthritis following a cognitive behavioral intervention. *Biofeedback Self Regul* 1995 Sep;20(3):259-68

Zachariae R, Kristensen JS, Hokland P, Ellegaard J, Metze E, Hokland M. Effect of psychological intervention in the form of relaxation and guided imagery on cellular immune function in normal healthy subjects. An overview. *Psychother Psychosom* 1990;54(1):32-9

PRAYER AND SPIRITUALITY

Bill-Harvey D, Rippey RM, Abeles M, Pfeiffer CA. Methods used by urban, low-income minorities to care for their arthritis. *Arthritis Care Res* 1989 Jun;2(2):60-4

Byrd RC . Positive therapeutic effects of intercessory prayer in a coronary care unit population. *South Med J* 1988 Jul;81(7):826-9

Koenig HG. Religious attitudes and practices of hospitalized medically ill older adults. *Int J Geriatr Psychiatry* 1998 Apr;13(4):213-24

Koenig HG, Larson DB. Use of hospital services, religious attendance, and religious affiliation. *South Med J* 1998 Oct;91(10):925-32

Matthews DA, Marlowe SM, McNutt FS. Beneficial effects of intercessory prayer ministry in patients with rheumatoid arthritis. *J General Intern Med* 1998;13(suppl)

Oman D, Reed D. Religion and mortality among the community-dwelling elderly. *Am J Public Health* 1998 Oct;88(10):1469-75

Orr RD, Isaac G. Religious variables are infrequently reported in clinical research. *Fam Medicine* 1992 24(8):602-6

Oxman TE, Freeman DH Jr, Manheimer ED. Lack of social participation or religious strength and comfort as risk factors for death after cardiac surgery in the elderly. *Psychosom Med* 1995 Jan-Feb;57(1):5-15

Pioro-Boisset M, Esdaile JM, Fitzcharles MA. Alternative medicine use in fibromyalgia syndrome [see comments] *Arthritis Care Res* 1996 Feb;9(1):13-7. Comment in: *Arthritis Care Res* 1996 Feb;9(1):1-2

Sicher F, Targ E, Moore D, Smith HS. A randomized double-blind study of the effect of distant healing in a population with advanced AIDS. Report of a small scale study. *West J Med* 1998 Dec;169(6):356-63

Sloan RP, Bagiella E, Powell T. Religion, spirituality, and medicine. *Lancet* 1999 Feb 20;353(9153):664-7

Strawbridge WJ, Cohen RD, Shema SJ, Kaplan GA. Frequent attendance at religious services and mortality over 28 years. *Am J Public Health* 1997 Jun;87(6):957-61

MOVING MEDICINE

Austin JHM, Ausubel P. Enhanced respiratory muscular function in normal adults after lessons in proprioceptive musculoskeletal education with exercises. *Chest* 1992;102:486-90

Dennis RJ. Functional reach improvement in normal older women after Alexander technique instruction. *J Gerontol* A Biol Sci Med Sci Jan 1999;54:M8-11

Fisher K. Early Experiences of a Multidisciplinary Pain Management Programme. *Holistic Medicine* 1988;3:47-56

Garfinkel MS, Singhal A, Katz WA, Allan DA, Reshetar R, Schumacher HR. Yoga for carpal tunnel syndrome. *JAMA* 1998; 280:1601-1603

Garfinkel MS, Schumacher HR Jr, Husain A, Levy M, Reshetar RA. Evaluation of a yoga based regimen for treatment of osteoarthritis in the hands. *Journal of Rheumatology* Dec 1994; 21:2341-43

Haslock I, Monroe, Nagaratha, Nagendra, Raghuram. Measuring the effects of yoga in rheumatoid arthritis. *British Journal of Rheumatology* 1994;33:787-88

Khumar SS, Kaur P, Kaur S. Effectiveness of Shavasana on depression among university students. *Indian Journal of Clinical Psychology* Sep 1993;20:82-87

Kirsteins AE, Dietz F, Hwang SM. Evaluating the safety and potential use of a weight-bearing exercise, Tai-Chi Chuan, for rheumatoid arthritis patients. *Am J Phys Med Rehabil* Jun 1991;70(3):P136-41

Sahasi G, Mohan D, Kacker C. Effectiveness of yogic techniques in the management of anxiety. *Journal of Personality and Clinical Studies* Mar 1989;5:51-55

Singh BB, Berman BM, Hadhazy VA, Creamer P. A pilot study of cognitive behavioral therapy in fibromyalgia. *Altern Ther Health Med* 1998;4(2):67-70

Witt P, MacKinnon J. A method to improve chest mobility of patients with chronic lung disease. *Physical Therapy* 1986;66:214-17

Wolf SL, Barnhart H, Kutner NG, et al. Reducing frailty and falls in older persons: an investigation of Tai Chi and computerized balance training. *J Am Geriatrics Soc* 1996;44:489-497

Wolfson LR, Whipple C, Derby, et al. Balance and strength training in older adults: Intervention gains and Tai Chi maintenance. *J Am Geriatrics Soc* 1996;44:498-506

Wood C. Mood change and perceptions of vitality: a comparison of the effects of relaxation, visualization and yoga. *J Royal Soc Med* 5-1993;86: 254-258

MASSAGE AND BODYWORK

Christensen, BV. Acupuncture treatment of severe knee osteoarthritis. A long-term study. *Acta Anaesthesiol Scand* 1992;36(6):519-25

DeLuze C, Bosia L, Zirbs A, Chantraine A, Vicher TL. Electroacupuncture in fibromyalgia: results of a controlled trial. *Br Med* J 1992;305:1249-52

Eisenberg DM, Davis R, Ettner S, Appel S, Wilkey S, Van Rampay M, Kessler RC. Trends in alternative medicine use in the United States, 1990-1997. *JAMA* 1998;280:1569 75

Field T, et al. Massage of pre-term newborns to improve growth and development. *Pediatric Nursing* 1987;13, 385-387

Field TM, Sunshine W, Hernandez-Reif, Quintino O, Schanberg S, Kuhn C, Burman I. Massage therapy effects on depression and somatic symptoms in chronic fatigue syndrome. *Journal of Chronic Fatigue Syndrome* 1997;3:43-51

Field TM, Hernandez-Reif M, Seligman S, Krasnegor J, Sunshine W. Juvenile rheumatoid arthritis: benefits from massage therapy. *Journal of Pediatric Psychology Proceedings.* 1997;22:607-617

Gordon A, Merenstein JH, D'Amica F, Hudgens D. The effects of therapeutic touch on patients with osteoarthritis of the knee. *J Fam Pract.* 1998 Oct;47(4):271-7

Hirschberg G. Skinfold tenderness and skinrolling massage in fibromyalgia. *J of Orthop Med* 1997; 19(3):77-82

Ironson G, T. Massage therapy is associated with enhancement of the immune system's cytotoxic capacity. *Inter J Neuroscience* 1996;84:205-217

Oleson T, Flocco W. Randomized controlled study of premenstrual symptoms treated with ear, hand, and foot reflexology. *Obstet Gynecol* 1993 Dec;82(6):906-11

Olson K, Hanson J. Using Reiki to manage pain: a preliminary report. *Cancer Prev Control.* 1997 Jun;1(2):108-13

Perry J, Jones MH, Thomas L. Functional evaluation of Rolfing in cerebral palsy. *Dev Med Child Neurol.* 1981;23(6):717-29

Rogers JS, Witt PL. The controversy of cranial bone motion. *J Orthop Sports Phys Ther.* 1997;26(2):95-103

Rogers JS, Witt PL, Gross MT, Hacke JD, Genova PA. Simultaneous palpation of the craniosacral rate at the head and feet: intrarater and interrater reliability and rate comparisons. *Phys Ther* 1998;78:1175-85

Rosa L, Rosa E, Sarner L, Barrnett S. A close look at therapeutic touch. *JAMA* 1998;279:1005-10

Sprott H, Franke S, Kluge H, Hein G. Pain treatment of fibromyalgia. *Rheumatol Int* 1998;18:35-5

Sunshine W, Field TM , Quintino O, Fierro K, Kuhn C, Burman I, Schanberg S. Fibromyalgia benefits from massage therapy and transcutaneous electrical stimulation. *J Clin Rheumatol.* 1996;2:18-22

Weinberg RS, Hunt VV. Effects of structural integration on state-trait anxiety. *J Clin Psychol* 1979;35:319-22

ACUPUNCTURE AND ACUPRESSURE

Allen JH, Rosa N, Schnyer, Sabrina K. The Efficacy of acupuncture in the treatment of major depression in women. *Psychological Science* 1998;9:397-401

Appiah R, Hiller S, Caspary L, Alexander K, Creutzig A. Treatment of primary Raynaud's syndrome with traditional Chinese acupuncture. *J Intern Med* 1997;241:119-24

Berman B, Lao L, et al. Efficacy of traditional Chinese acupuncture in the treatment of symptomatic knee osteoathritis: a pilot study. *Osteoarthritis and Cartilage*. 1995;3:139-142

Chan J, Carr I, Mayberry JF. The role of acupuncture in the treatment of irritable bowel syndrome: a pilot study. *Hepatogastroenterology* 1997;44:1328-30

Christensen, BV, Juhl IU, Vilbek H, Bulow HH, Dreijer NC, Rasmussen HF. Acupuncture treatment of severe knee osteoarthrosis. A long-term study. *Acta Anaesthesiol Scand* 1992;36:519-25

David J, Townsend S, Sathananthan, Kriss S, Dore C. The effect of acupuncture on patients with rheumatoid arthritis: a randomized placebo controlled crossover study. *Arthritis Rheum* 1998;41(suppl):S316

DeLuze C, Bosia L, Zirbs A, Chantraine A, Vicher TL. Electroacupuncture in fibromyalgia: results of a controlled study. *Br Med J* 1992;305:1249-52

Ernst E, White AR. Acupuncture for back pain: a meta-analysis of randomized controlled trials. *Arch Intern Med*. 1998;158:2235-41

Jerner B, Skogh M, Vahlquist A. A controlled trial of acupuncture in psoriasis: no convincing effect. *Acta Derm Venereol* 1997;77:154-6

Kurland HD. Treatment of headache pain with auto-acupressure. *Dis Nerv Syst* 1976;37:127-9

Lautenschlager J. Acupuncture in treatment of inflammatory rheumatic diseases. *Z Rheumatol* 1997;56:L8-20

List T, Lundeberg T, Lundstrong I, Lindstrom F, Ravald N. The effect of acupuncture in the treatment of patients with primary Sjogren's syndrome. A controlled study. *Acta Odontol Scand* 1998;56:95-9

NIH (National Institutes of Health) Consensus Development Statement on Acupuncture. David J. Ramsay, DM, DPhil., Marjorie A. Bowman, MD, M.P.A , Philip E. Greenman, DO, FAAO, Stephen P. Jiang, ACSW, Lawrence H. Kushi, ScD, Keh-Ming Lin, MD, MPH, Susan Leeman, PhD, Daniel E. Moerman, PhD, Sidney H. Schnoll, MD, PhD, Marcellus Walker, MD, Christine Waternaux, PhD. Nov 3-5 1997

Sprott H, Franke S, Kluge H, Hein G. Pain treatment of fibromyalgia by acupuncture [letter]. *Rheumatol Int* 1998;18:35-6

Sprott H, Franke S, Dluge H, Hein G. Pain treatment of fibromyalgia by acupuncture. *Arthritis Rheum* 1996;39(suppl):S91

MISCELLANEOUS THERAPIES

Beckerman H, de Bie RA, Bouter LM, De Cuyper HJ, Oostendorp RA. The efficacy of laser therapy for musculoskeletal and skin disorders: a criteria-based meta-analysis of randomized clinical trials. *Phys Ther* 1992;72:483-91

Bulow PM, Jensen H; Danneskiold-Samsoe B. Low power Ga-Al-As laser treatment of painful osteoarthritis of the knee. A double-blind placebo-controlled study. *Scand J Rehabil Med* 1994;26:155-9

Chang YH, Bliven. Anti-arthritic effect of bee venom. *Agents Actions* 1979;9:205-11

Eiseman JL, von Bredow J, Alvares AP. Effect of honeybee (*Apis mellifera*) venom on the course of adjuvant-induced arthritis and depression of drug metabolism in the rat. *Biochem Pharmacol* 1982;31:1139-46

Hall J, Clarke AK, Elvins DM, Ring EF. Low level laser therapy is ineffective in the management of rheumatoid arthritic finger joints. *Br J Rheumatol* 1994;33:142-7

Heussler JK, Hinchey G, Margiotta E, Quinn R, Butler P, Martin J, Sturgess AD. A double blind randomised trial of low power laser treatment in rheumatoid arthritis. *Ann Rheum Dis* 1993;52:703-6

Johannsen F, Hauschild B, Remig L, Johnsen V,Petersen M, Bieler T. Low energy laser therapy in rheumatoid arthritis. *Scan J Rheumatol* 1994;23:145-7

Trock DH, Bollet AJ, Dyer RH, Fielding LP, Miner WK, Markoll R. A double blind trial of the clinical effects of pulsed electromagnetic fields in osteoarthritis. *J Rheumatol* 1993;20:456-60. Comment in: *J Rheumatol* 1993;20:2166-7

Trock DH, Bollet AJ, Markoll R. The effect of pulsed electromagnetic fields in the treatment of osteoarthritis of the knee and cervical spine. *J Rheumatol* 1994;21:1903

Vallbona C, Hazlewood CF, Jurida G. Response of pain to static magnetic fields in postpolio patients: a double-blind pilot study. *Arch Phys Med Rehabil* 1997 ;78:1200-3. Comment in *Arch Phys Med Rehabil* 1998;79:469-70

Walker WR, Keats DM. An investigation of the therapeutic value of the 'copper bracelet'- dermal assimilation of copper in arthritic/rheumatoid conditions. *Agents Actions* 1976;6:454-9

Weinberger A, Nyska A, Giler S. Treatment of experimental inflammatory synovitis with continuous magnetic field. *Isr J Med Sci* 1996;32:1197

Weintraub MI. Noninvasive laser neurolysis in carpal tunnel syndrome. *Muscle Nerve* 1997;20:1029-31

Weintraub, MI. Magnetic biostimulation in painful diabetic peripheral neuropathy: a novel intervention. *Am J Pain Management* 1999;9:9-18

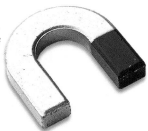

Zizic TM, Hoffman KC, Holt PA, et al. The treatment of osteoarthritis of the knee with pulsed electrical stimulation. *J Rheumatol* 1995;22:1757-61

Zurier RB, et al. Effect of bee venom on experimental arthritis. *Ann Rheum Dis.* 1973;32:466-70

FOOD AND ARTHRITIS

Belch JJ, Ansell D, Madhok R, O'Dowd A, Sturrock RD. Effects of altering dietary essential fatty acids on requirements for non-steroidal anti-inflammatory drugs in patients with rheumatoid arthritis: a double blind placebo controlled study. *Ann Rheum Dis* 1998;47:96-104

Bjarnason I, Williams P, So A, Zanelli GD, Levi AJ, Gumpel JM, Peters TJ, Ansell B. Intestinal permeability and inflammation in rheumatoid arthritis: effects of non-steroidal anti-inflammatory drugs. *Lancet* 1984;2(8413):1171-4

Childers NF. A relationship of arthritis to the Solanacea (nightshades). *Journal of the International Academy of Preventive Medicine* 1982 Vol VII, No. 3

Darlington LG, Ramsey NW. Review of dietary therapy for rheumatoid arthritis [see comments] Rheumatology Unit, Epsom General Hospital, Surrey. *Br J Rheumatol* 1993;32:507-14. Comment in *Br J Rheumatol* 1993;32:1030

Darlington LG, Ramsey NW, Mansfield JR. Placebo-controlled, blind study of dietary manipulation therapy in rheumatoid arthritis. *Lancet* 1986;1(8475):236-8

DiGiacomo RA, Kremer JM, Shah DM. Fish-oil dietary supplementation in patients with Raynaud's phenomenon: a double-blind, controlled, prospective study. *Am J Med* 1989;86:158-64

Kjeldsen-Kragh J, Haugen M, Borchgrevink CF, Laerum E, Eek M, Mowinkel P, Hovi K, Forre O. Controlled trial of fasting and one-year vegetarian diet in rheumatoid arthritis. *Lancet.* 1991;338(8772):899-902. Comment in *Lancet* 1991;338(8776):1209-10. Comment in *Lancet* 1992;339(8802):1177

Kjeldsen-Kragh J, Haugen M, Borchgrevink CF, Forre O. Vegetarian diet for patients with rheumatoid arthritis — status: two years after introduction of the diet. *Clin Rheumatol* 1994;13:475-82

Kremer JM, Lawrence DA, Jubiz W, DiGiacomo R, Rynes R, Bartholomew LE, Sherman M. Dietary fish oil and olive oil supplementation in patients with rheumatoid arthritis. Clinical and immunologic effects. *Arthritis Rheum* 1990;33:810-20

Leventhal LJ, Boyce EG, Zurier RB. Treatment of rheumatoid arthritis with gammalinolenic acid. *Ann Intern Med* 1993;119:867-73

Nenonen MT, Helve TA, Rauma AL, Hanninen OO. Uncooked, lactobacilli-rich, vegan food and rheumatoid arthritis. *Br J Rheumatol* 1998;37:274-81

Panush RS, Stroud RM, Webster EM. Food-induced (allergic) arthritis. inflammatory arthritis exacerbated by milk. *Arthritis Rheum* 1986;29:220-6

Panush RS, Carter RL, Katz P, Kowsari B, Longley S, Finnie S. Diet therapy for rheumatoid arthritis. *Arthritis Rheum* 1983;26:462-71

Parke AL, et al. Rheumatoid arthritis and food: a case study. *Br Med J* (Clin Res Ed) 1981;282:2027-9

Ratner D, et al. Juvenile rheumatoid arthritis and milk allergy. *J R Soc Med.* 1985;78:410-3

Skoldstam L, Magnusson KE. Fasting, intestinal permeability, and rheumatoid arthritis. *Rheum Dis Clin North Am* 1991;17(2):363-71

Skoldstam L, Larsson L, Lindstrom FD. Effect of fasting and lactovegetarian diet on rheumatoid arthritis. *Scand J Rheumatol* 1979;8(4):249-55

van de Laar MA, van der Korst JK. Food intolerance in rheumatoid arthritis. I. A double blind, controlled trial of the clinical effects of elimination of milk allergens and azo dyes. *Ann Rheum Dis* 1992;51(3):298-302. Comment in *Ann Rheum Dis* 1993;52(1):88

Ammon HP, Safayhi H, Mack T, Sabieraj J. Mechanism of antiinflammatory actions of curcumine and boswellic acids. *J Ethnopharmacol* 1993;38(2-3):113-9

Barnett ML, Kremer JM, St. Clair EW, et al. Treatment of rheumatoid arthritis with oral type II collagen. Results of a multicenter, double-blind, placebo-controlled trial. *Arthritis Rheum* 1998;41:290-7

Belch JJ, Ansell D, Madhok R, O'Dowd A, Sturrock RD. Effects of altering dietary essential fatty acids on requirements for non-steroidal anti-inflammatory drugs in patients with rheumatoid arthritis: a double blind placebo controlled study. *Ann Rheum Dis* 1988;47:96-104

Bensoussan A, Talley NJ, Hing M, Menzies R, Guo A, Ngu M. Treatment of irritable bowel syndrome with Chinese herbal medicine: a randomized controlled trial. *JAMA* 1998;280:1585-9

Blankenhorn G. Klinische Wirksamkeit von Spondyvit (vitamin E) bei aktivierten Arthrosen. Eine multicentrische placebokontrollierte Doppelblindstudie. [Clinical effectiveness of Spondyvit (vitamin E) in activated arthroses. A multicenter placebo-controlled double-blind study] *Z Orthop* 1986;124(3):340-3

Blotman F, Maheu E, Wulwik A, Caspard H, Lopez A. Efficacy and safety of avocado/soybean unsaponifiables in the treatment of symptomatic osteoarthritis of the knee and hip. A prospective, multicenter, three month, randomized, double-blind, placebo-controlled trial. *Rev Rhum Engl Ed* 1997;64:825-34

Boumediene K, Felisaz N, Bogdanowicz P, Galera P; Guillou GB, Pujol JP. Avocado/soya unsaponifiables enhance the expression of transforming growth factor beta1 and beta2 in cultured articular chondrocytes. *Arthritis Rheum* 1999;42:148-56

Bradley JD, Flusser D, Katz BP, Schumacher HR Jr, Brandt KD, Chambers MA, Zonay LJ. A randomized, double blind, placebo controlled trial of intravenous loading with S-adenosylmethionine (SAM) followed by oral SAM therapy in patients with knee osteoarthritis. *J Rheumatol* 1994;21(5):905-11

Bressa GM. S-adenosyl-l-methionine (SAMe) as antidepressant: meta-analysis of clinical studies. *Acta Neurol Scand Suppl* 1994;154:7-14

Chopra A, Patwardhan B, Lavin P, Chitre D. A randomized placebo-controlled trial of an herbal Ayurvedic formulation in patients with active rheumatoid arthritis [abstract]. *Arthritis Rheum* 1996:39(suppl):S283

Chopra A, Lavin P, Chitre D, Patwardhan B, Polisson R. A clinical study of an Ayurvedic (Asian Indian) medicine in OA knees [abstract]. *Arthritis Rheum* 1998;41(suppl):S198

Chou CT, Chang SC. The inhibitory effect of common traditional anti-rheumatic herb formulas on prostaglandin E and interleukin 2 in vitro: a comparative study with *Tripterygium wilfordii. J Ethnopharmacol* 1998;62:167-71

Chrubasik S, Enderlein W, Bauer R, Grabner W. Evicence for antirheumatic effectiveness of Herba Urticae dioicae in acute arthritis: a pilot study. *Phytomedicine* 1997;4(2):105-8

Chrubasik S, Wink M. Traditional herbal therapy for the treatment of rheumatic pain: Preparations from Devil's Claw and stinging nettle. *Pain Digest* 1998 Aug:94-101

Clark WF, Parbtani A, Huff MW, Spanner E, de Salis H, Chin-Yee I, Philbrick DJ, Holub BJ. Flaxseed: a potential treatment for lupus nephritis. *Kidney Int* 1995;48(2):475-80

Clemmensen OJ, Siggaard-Andersen J, Worm AM, Stahl D, Frost F, Bloch I. Psoriatic arthritis treated with oral zinc sulphate. *Br J Dermatol* 1980;103:411-5

Cohen A, Goldman J. Bromelains therapy in rheumatoid arthritis. *Penn Med J* 1964;67:27-30

Cox IM, Campbell MJ, Dowson D. Red blood cell magnesium and chronic fatigue syndrome. *Lancet* 1991;337(8744):757-60

Nature's Remedies continued

Csuka ME, Taylor ML, Tapal M, Madigan, TJ, Gardner J, Tonellato P. Randomized double blind placebo controlled trial comparing melatonin to placebo in the treatment of fibromyalgia [abstract]. *Arthritis Rheum* 1998;41(suppl):S258

da Camara CC, Dowless GV. Glucosamine sulfate for osteoarthritis. *Ann Pharmacother* 1998;32(5):580-7. Comment in *Ann Pharmacother* 1998;32(5):602-3

D'Angelo L, Grimaldi R, Caravaggi M, Marcoli M, Perucca E, Lecchini S, Frigo GM, Crema A. A double-blind, placebo-controlled clinical study on the effect of a standardized ginseng extract on psychomotor performance in healthy volunteers. *J Ethnopharmacol* 1986;16(1):15-22

Davis RH, Leitner MG, Russo JM, Byrne ME. Wound healing. Oral and topical activity of Aloe vera. *J Am Podiatr Med Assoc* 1989;79:559-62

Diehl HW, May EL. Cetyl myristoleate isolated from Swiss albino mice: an apparent protective agent against adjuvant arthritis in rats. *J Pharm Sci* 1994;83:296-9

DiGiacomo RA, Kremer JM, Shah DM. Fish-oil dietary supplementation in patients with Raynaud's phenomenon: a double-blind, controlled, prospective study. *Am J Med* 1989;86(2):158-64

Dowling EA, Redondo DR, Branch JD, Jones S, McNabb G, Williams MH. Effect of Eleutherococcus senticosus on submaximal and maximal exercise performance. *Med Sci Sports Exerc* 1996;28(4):482-9

Eberhardt R, Zwingers T, Hofmann R. DMSO bei Patienten mit aktivierter Gonarthrose. Eine doppelblinde, plazebokontrollierte Phase-III-Studie. [DMSO in patients with active gonarthrosis. A double-blind placebo controlled phase III study] *Fortschr Med* 1995;113(31):446-50

Ernst E. Johanniskraut zur antidepressiven Therapie. [St. John's wort as antidepressive therapy] *Fortschr Med* 1995;113(25):354-5

Fava M, Giannelli A, Rapisarda V, Patralia A, Guaraldi GP. Rapidity of onset of the antidepressant effect of parenteral S-adenosyl- L-methionine. *Psychiatry Res* 1995;56:295-7

Fracp RL, Travers, Rennie GC, Newnham RX. Boron and arthritis: the results of double-blind study. *J Nutritional Med* 1990;1:127-32

Fujiki H, Suganuma M, Okabe S, Sueoka E, Suga K, Imai K, Nakachi K, Kimura S. Mechanistic findings of green tea as cancer preventive for humans. *Proc Soc Exp Biol Med* 1999;220:225-8

Hanley D, Solomon W, Saffrant B, Davis R. The evaluation of natural substances in the treatment of adjuvant arthritis. *J Am Podiatry Assoc* 1982;72:276-84

Haqqi TM, Anthony DD, Gupta S, Ahmad N, Lee M, Kumar GK, Mukhtar H. Prevention of collagen-induced arthritis in mice by a polyphenolic fraction from green tea. *Proc Natl Acad Sci U S A* 1999;96:4524-9

Hauselmann HJ, Caravatti M, Seifert B, Wang K, Bruckner P, Stucki G, Michel BA. Can collagen type II sustain a methotrexate-induced therapeutic effect in patients with long-standing rheumatoid arthritis? A double-blind, randomized trial. *Br J Rheumatol* 1998;37:1110-7

Heggers JP, Kucukcelebi A, Listengarten D, Stabenau J, Ko F, Broemeling LD, Robson MC, Winters WD. Beneficial effect of aloe on wound healing in an excisional wound model. *J Altern Complement Med* 1996;2:271-7

Heinle K, Adam A, Gradl M, Wiseman M, Adam. Selenkonzentration in den Erythrozyten bei Patienten mit rheumatoider Arthritis. Klinische und laborchemische Entzundungszeichen unter Supplementierung mit Selen. [Selenium concentration in erythrocytes of patients with rheumatoid arthritis. Clinical and laboratory chemistry infection markers during administration of selenium]. *Med Klin* 1997;92 (Suppl 3):29-31

Hunt CD, Idso JP. Dietary boron as a physiological regulator of the normal inflammatory response: a review and current research progress. J *Trace Elements Experimental Med.* [In Press]

JAMA. Copper boosts activity of anti-inflammatory drugs. *JAMA.* 1974; 229(10)

Jamieson DD, Duffield PH. Positive interaction of ethanol and kava resin in mice. *Clin Exp Pharmacol Physiol* 1990;17(7):509-14

Joe B, Rao UJ, Lokesh BR Presence of an acidic glycoprotein in the serum of arthritic rats: modulation by capsaicin and curcumin. *Mol Cell Biochem* 1997;169:125-34

Jonas WB, Rapoza CP, Blair WF. The effect of niacinamide on osteoarthritis: a pilot study. *Inflamm Res* 1996;45(7):330

Jordan JM, Luta G, DeRoos A, Kohlmeier L, Renner JB. Naturally-occurring anti-oxidants may prevent knee osteoarthritis [abstract]. *Arthritis Rheum* 1998;41(suppl):S133

Jung F, Mrowietz C, Kiesewetter H, Wenzel E. Effect of Ginkgo biloba on fluidity of blood and peripheral microcirculation in volunteers. *Arzneimittelforschung* 1990;40(5):589-93

Kelly GS. The role of glucosamine sulfate and chondroitin sulfate in the treatment of degenerative joint disease. *Altern Med Rev* 1998;3(1):27-39

Khalkhali-Ellis Z, Moore TL, Hendrix MJ. Reduced levels of testosterone and dehydroepiandrosterone sulphate in the serum and synovial fluid of juvenile rheumatoid arthritis patients correlates with disease severity. *Clin Exp Rheumatol* 1998;16(6):753-6

Kinzler E, Kromer J, Lehmann E. [Effect of a special kava extract in patients with anxiety-, tension-, and excitation states of non-psychotic genesis. Double blind study with placebos over 4 weeks]. *Arzneimittelforschung* 1991;41(6):584-8

Korszun A, Papadopoulous E, Engleberg NC, Haus E, Lundeen L, Smolensky M, Demitrack MA, Crofford LJ. Circanian rhythms of melatonin and cortisol in women with fibromyalgia (FM) and chronic fatigue syndrome (CFS). *Arthritis Rheum* 1997;40(suppl):S43

Kremer JM, Lawrence DA, Petrillo GF, Litts LL, Mullaly PM, Rynes RI, Stocker RP, Parhami N, Greenstein NS, Fuchs BR et al. Effects of high-dose fish oil on rheumatoid arthritis after stopping nonsteroidal antiinflammatory drugs. Clinical and immune correlates. *Arthritis Rheum* 1995;38(8):1107-14

Kulkarni RR, Patki PS, Jog VP, Gandage SG, Patwardhan B. Treatment of osteoarthritis with a herbomineral formulation: a double-blind, placebo-controlled, cross-over study. J *Ethnopharmacol* 1991;33:91-5

Lau CS, Morley KD, Belch JJ. Effects of fish oil supplementation on non-steroidal anti-inflammatory drug requirement in patients with mild rheumatoid arthritis — a double-blind placebo controlled study. *Br J Rheumatol* 1993;32:982-9

Leathwood PD, Chauffard F, Heck E, Munoz-Box R. Aqueous extract of valerian root (*Valeriana officinalis L.*) improves sleep quality in man. *Pharmacol Biochem Behav* 1982;17(1):65-71

Nature's Remedies continued

Leventhal LJ, Boyce EG, Zurier RB. Treatment of rheumatoid arthritis with gammalinolenic acid. *Ann Intern Med* 1993;119:867-73. Comment in *Ann Intern Med* 1994;120:692

Lewis WH, Zenger VE, Lynch RG. No adaptogen response of mice to ginseng and Eleutherococcus infusions. *J Ethnopharmacol* 1983;8:209-14

Lipsky PE, Tao XL. A potential new treatment for rheumatoid arthritis: thunder god vine. *Semin Arthritis Rheum* 1997;26:713-23

Machtey I, Ouaknine L. Tocopherol in osteoarthritis: a controlled pilot study. *J Am Geriatr Soc* 1978;26:328-30

Maheu E, Mazieres B, Valat JP, Loyau G, Le Loet X, Bourgeois P, Grouin JM, Rozenberg S. Symptomatic efficacy of avocado/soybean unsaponifiables in the treatment of osteoarthritis of the knee and hip: a prospective, randomized, double-blind, placebo-controlled, multicenter clinical trial with a six-month treatment period and a two-month followup demonstrating a persistent effect [see comments] *Arthritis Rheum* 1998;41:81-91. Comment in *Arthritis Rheum* 1998;41:1705

Mantzioris E, James MJ, Gibson RA, Cleland LG. Dietary substitution with an alpha-linolenic acid-rich vegetable oil increases eicosapentaenoic acid concentrations in tissues. *Am J Clin Nutr* 1994;59:1304-9

McAlindon TE, Felson DT, Zhang Y, Hannan MT, Aliabadi P, Weissman B, Rush D, Wilson PW, Jacques P. Relation of dietary intake and serum levels of vitamin D to progression of osteoarthritis of the knee among participants in the Framingham Study. *Ann Intern Med* 1996;125:353-9

McAlindon TE, et al. Do antioxidant micronutrients protect against the development and progression of knee osteoarthritis? *Arthritis Rheum* 1996;39:648-56

McCarthy GM, Marty DJ. Effect of topical capsaicin in the therapy of painful osteoarthritis of the hands. *J Rheumatol* 1992;19:604-7

Melchart D, Linde K, Worku F, Sarkady L, Holzmann M, Jurcic K, Wagner H. Results of five randomized studies on the immunomodulatory activity of preparations of Echinacea. *J Altern Complement Med* 1995;1:145-60

Miller LG. Herbal medicinals: selected clinical considerations focusing on known or potential drug-herb interactions. *Arch Intern Med* 1998;158:2200-11

Moore RD, Morton JI. Diminished inflammatory joint disease in MRL/1pr mice ingesting dimethylsulfoxide (DMSO) or methylsulfonylmethane (MSM). *Immunopathology 1985;1:692-697*

Morton JI, Siegel BV. Effects of oral dimethyl sulfoxide and dimethyl sulfone on murine autoimmune lymphoproliferative disease. *Proc Soc Exp Biol Med* 1986;183:227-30

Muller-Fassbender H. Rheumazentrum Bad Abbach, II Medizinische Klinik, Bad Abbach, [Double-blind clinical trial of S-adenosylmethionine versus ibuprofen in the treatment of osteoarthritis]. *Am J Med* 1987;83(5A):81-3

Newnham RE. Essentiality of boron for healthy bones and joints. *Environ Health Perspect* 1994;102 Suppl 7:83-5

Nielsen. Effect of dietary boron on mineral, estrogen and testosterone metabolism in postmenopausal women. *FASEB J* 1987;1:394-97.

Nordstrom DC, Honkanen VE, Nasu Y, Antila E, Friman C, Konttinen YT. Alpha-linolenic acid in the treatment of rheumatoid arthritis. A double-blind, placebo-controlled and randomized study: flaxseed vs. safflower seed. *Rheumatol Int* 1995;14:231-4

Norton SA. Herbal medicines in Hawaii from tradition to convention. *Hawaii Med J* 1998;57(1):382-6

Obertreis B, Giller K, Teucher T, Behnke B, Schmitz H. [Anti-inflammatory effect of Urtica dioica folia extract in comparison to caffeic malic acid.] Arzneimittelforschung 1996;46:52-6

O'Dell JR, McGivern JP, Kay HD, Klassen LW. Improved survival in murine lupus as the result of selenium supplementation. *Clin Exp Immunol* 1988;73:322-7

O'Hara M, Kiefer D, Farrell K, Kemper K. A review of 12 commonly used medicinal herbs. *Arch Fam Med* 1998;7:523-36

Petri M, Lahita R, Schiff M, Ginzler E, van Vollenhoven R. Results of the GL701 DHEA multi-center steroid-sparing SLE study [abstract]. Lupus 1998;7(Supp):120

Petri M, Vu D, Omura A, Yuen J, Selhub J, Rosenberg I, Roubenoff R. Effectiveness of B-vitamin therapy in reducing plasma total homocysteine in patients with systemic lupus erythematosus (SLE) [abstract]. *Arthritis Rheum* 1998;41(suppl):S241

Press J, Phillip M, Neumann L, Barak R, Segev Y, Abu-Shakra M, Buskila D. Normal melatonin levels in patients with fibromyalgia syndrome. *J Rheumatol* 1998;25:551-5

Qiu GX, Gao SN, Giacovelli G, Rovati L, Setnikar I. Efficacy and safety of glucosamine sulfate versus ibuprofen in patients with knee osteoarthritis. *Arzneimittelforschung* 1998;48:469-74

Rains C, Bryson HM. Topical capsaicin. A review of its pharmacological properties and therapeutic potential in post-herpetic neuralgia, diabetic neuropathy and osteoarthritis. *Drugs Aging* 1995;7:317-28

Russell IJ, Michalek JE, Flechas JD, Abraham GE. Treatment of fibromyalgia syndrome with Super Malic: a randomized, double blind, placebo controlled, crossover pilot study. *J Rheumatol* 1995;22:953-8

Sander O; Herborn G; Rau R. [Is H15 (resin extract of *Boswellia serrata*, "incense") a useful supplement to established drug therapy of chronic polyarthritis? Results of a double-blind pilot study] *Z Rheumatol* 1998;57:11-6

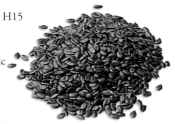

Sandoval-Chacon M, et al. Antiinflammatory actions of cat's claw: the role of NF-kappaB [In Process Citation]. *Ailment Pharmacol Ther* 1998;12:1279-89

Scherak O, Kolarz G, Schodl C, Blankenhorn G. Hochdosierte Vitamin-E-Therapie bei Patienten mit aktivierter Arthrose. [High dosage vitamin E therapy in patients with activated arthrosis] *Z Rheumatol* 1990;49:369-73

Scherbel AL, Lawrence J, McCormack, Layle JK. Further observations on the effect of dimethyl sulfoxide in patients with generalized scleroderma (progressive systemic sclerosis). *Annals NY Acad Sci.* 1968, pp. 613-629

Schmitz M, Jackel M. [Comparative study for assessing quality of life of patients with exogenous sleep disorders (temporary sleep onset and sleep interruption disorders) treated with a hops-valarian preparation and a benzodiazepine drug]. *Wien Med Wochenschr* 1998;148(13):291-8

Sieper J, Kary S, Sorensen H, et al. Oral type II collagen treatment in early rheumatoid arthritis. A double-blind, placebo-controlled, randomized trial. *Arthritis Rheum* 1996;39:41-51

Simkin PA. Oral zinc sulphate in rheumatoid arthritis. *Lancet* 1976;2(7985):539-42

Sorenson JR, Hangarter W. Treatment of rheumatoid and degenerative diseases with copper complexes: a review with emphasis on copper-salicylate. *Inflammation* 1977;2:217-38

Srivastava KC, Mustafa T. Ginger (*Zingiber officinale*) in rheumatism and musculoskeletal disorders. *Med Hypotheses* 1992;39:342-8

Nature's Remedies continued

Tao XL, Sun Y, Dong Y, Xiao YL, Hu DW, Shi YP, Zhu QL, Dai H, Zhang NZ . A prospective, controlled, double-blind, cross-over study of *tripterygium wilfodii hook F* in treatment of rheumatoid arthritis. *Chin Med J (Engl)* 1989;102(5):327-32

Tarp U, Overvad K, Hansen JC, Thorling EB. Low selenium level in severe rheumatoid arthritis. *Scand J Rheumatol* 1985;14(2):97-101

Taussig SJ; Batkin S. Bromelain, the enzyme complex of pineapple (*Ananas comosus*) and its clinical application. An update. *J Ethnopharmacol* 1988;22(2):191-203

Trentham DE, Dynesius-Trentham RA, Orav EJ, et al. Effects of oral administration of type II collagen on rheumatoid arthritis. *Science* 1993;261(5129):1727-30

Uebelhart D, Thonar EJ, Delmas PD, Chantraine A, Vignon E. Effects of oral chondroitin sulfate on the progression of knee osteoarthritis: a pilot study. *Osteoarthritis Cartilage* 1998;6 (Suppl A):39-46

Van Vollenhoven RF, Morabito LM, Engleman EG, McGuire JL. Treatment of systemic lupus erythematosus with dehydroepiandrosterone: 50 patients treated up to 12 months. *J Rheumatol* 1998;25:285-9

Verbruggen G, Goemaere S, Veys EM. Chondroitin sulfate: S/DMOAD (structure/disease modifying anti-osteoarthritis drug) in the treatment of finger joint OA. *Osteoarthritis Cartilage* 1998;6 (Suppl A):37-8

Walker WR, Keats DM. An investigation of the therapeutic value of the 'copper bracelet'– dermal assimilation of copper in arthritic/rheumatoid conditions. *Agents Actions* 1976;6:454-9

Weisburger JH. Tea and health: the underlying mechanisms. *Proc Soc Exp Biol Med* 1999;220:271-5

Whitehouse LW, Znamirowska M, Paul CJ. Devil's claw (*Harpagophytum procumbens*): no evidence for anti-inflammatory activity in the treatment of arthritic disease. *Can Med Assoc J* 1983;129:249-51

Wikner J, Hirsch U, Wetterberg L, Rojdmark S. Fibromyalgia — a syndrome associated with decreased nocturnal melatonin secretion. *Clin Endocrinol* (Oxf) 1998;49:179-83

The Arthritis Foundation is the only national, voluntary health organization that works for all people affected by any of the 100-plus forms of arthritis or related diseases. Volunteers in chapters nationwide help to support research, professional and community education programs, services for people with arthritis, government advocacy on behalf of people with arthritis, and fund-raising activities.

The American Juvenile Arthritis Organization (AJAO), a council of the Arthritis Foundation, focuses its efforts on the problems and issues related to arthritis and similar conditions in children. It is composed of children, parents, health professionals, teachers and others who are concerned specifically about juvenile arthritis.

The goal of the Arthritis Foundation is two-fold: to support research to find the cure for and prevention of arthritis, and to improve the quality of life for those affected by arthritis. Public contributions enable the Arthritis Foundation to fulfill this mission. The Arthritis Foundation is the largest non-government supporter of arthritis-related research in the United States. In fact, at least 80 cents of every dollar contributed to the Arthritis Foundation helps fund the research, programs and services that make a difference in people's lives.

Research holds the key to future cures for and preventions of arthritis, but it takes time for researchers to make substantial progress. The good news is your condition doesn't have to rob you of the activities you enjoy most until those cures are found. The Arthritis Foundation believes it is equally important to improve the quality of life for people with arthritis *today*, which is why chapters offer information, programs and services to communities nationwide.

The Arthritis Foundation has more than 150 offices in the United States, so your road to living successfully with arthritis may be just a phone call away. Many chapters offer services such as those described in the following sections. Check your local phone book or call 800/283-7800 to find the Arthritis Foundation chapter nearest you and learn what programs and services it offers.

MEDICAL AND SELF-CARE PROGRAMS

Taking care of yourself physically is an important part of living well with arthritis or a related condition. The first step in that process is to get an early and accurate diagnosis from a physician. The Arthritis Foundation chapter in your area may offer the following programs and services to help further your efforts to take care of yourself.

Physician Referral

Working with a physician who is knowledgeable about arthritis is the key to a successful treatment program. Most Arthritis Foundation offices can provide you with a list of doctors in your area who specialize in the evaluation and treatment of arthritis and arthritis-related diseases.

Exercise Programs

Regular exercise is one of the most important steps in controlling your arthritis. You don't need to work out to the point of exhaustion to benefit from exercise. Every bit of activity is good for you physically and emotionally. These exercise programs are designed specifically for people with arthritis, and are led by specially trained instructors.

Joint Efforts. This arthritis movement program teaches gentle, undemanding movement exercises to help you maintain or regain your range of motion, even if you use a walker or wheelchair. Joint Efforts can also help decrease your pain, stiffness and depression.

PACE (People with Arthritis Can Exercise). You can increase your joint flexibility and range of motion and help maintain muscle strength using the gentle activities found in the Arthritis Foundation exercise program PACE. It can help you no matter your fitness level. Two videotapes that show basic and advanced levels of the program are available from your local Arthritis Foundation chapter for preview or for practice at home.

Arthritis Foundation Aquatics Program. This water exercise program was originally co-developed by the Arthritis Foundation and the YMCA. You can increase your muscle strength and endurance with this water exercise program. The water's buoyancy allows you to exercise without straining your joints.

EDUCATIONAL COURSES

If you live with a chronic condition like arthritis, taking an active role in your health care is especially important. Call your local Arthritis Foundation chapter to learn if the following classes are offered in your area.

Arthritis Foundation Self-Help Courses.

Gain the knowledge, skills and confidence needed to actively manage your condition. Courses focus on proper exercises, medications, relaxation techniques, pain and fatigue management, nutrition, and other relevant topics. Whether you have arthritis, fibromyalgia or lupus, one of the three different curriculums can help. Classes meet once weekly for six or seven weeks.

Bone Up On Arthritis

Learn much of the same information that is taught in Arthritis Foundation Self-Help Courses, with this self-study audio tape program. It is a good option for learning more about arthritis if a Self-Help Course isn't available in your area.

In Control

This program is another good option if a Self-Help Course isn't available in your area. Six lessons are presented on videotape and supplemented by a workbook and audio tapes.

RELIABLE INFORMATION AT YOUR FINGERTIPS

You know the adage: Knowledge is power. In addition to the classes and programs listed above, the Arthritis Foundation has information available in a variety of formats. With so many options for learning, you're sure to find just the information you need.

Information Hotline

The Arthritis Foundation is *the* expert on arthritis, and is only a phone call away. Call toll-free at 800/283-7800 for automated information on arthritis 24 hours a day. Trained volunteers and staff are also available at your local chapter to answer questions or send you a list of physicians in your area who specialize in arthritis.

Arthritis Foundation Web Site

If you're computer savvy and enjoy surfing the Internet, learn about arthritis 24 hours a day via the Arthritis Foundation's site on the World Wide Web. Check out http://www.arthritis.org for information on programs and services, publications, local chapter activities and more.

Publications

A number of publications are available to educate you and your family about important issues such as medications, exercise, diet and other day-to-day considerations.

Booklets. You can learn about arthritis-related conditions, medications and caring for yourself with the more than 60 booklets and brochures published by the Arthritis Foundation. Single copies are available from your local chapter free of charge. Call your local chapter or 800/283-7800 for a listing of available booklets.

Arthritis Today. This award-winning bi-monthly magazine gives you the latest information on research, new treatments and tips from experts and readers to help you manage your condition. Each issue also includes a variety of helpful articles to make your life with arthritis easier and more rewarding. A one-year subscription to *Arthritis Today* is yours free when you become a member of the Arthritis Foundation. Annual membership is $20 and helps fund research to find cures for arthritis. Call 800/933-0032 for membership and subscription information. *Arthritis Today* is also available nationwide on the newsstand, so look for it in your local bookstore.

Books. Self-care books are available from the Arthritis Foundation to help you learn more about your condition and how to manage it. Check your local bookstores, contact your local Arthritis Foundation chapter or call 800/207-8633 for available titles.

Audiovisual libraries

Many Arthritis Foundation chapters have audio and videotapes available for purchase or loan. Topics range from exercise to relaxation, and will vary from one chapter to another. Call your local chapter for a list of titles and prices.

REMEMBER THE ARTHRITIS FOUNDATION IN YOUR WILL

The mission of the Arthritis Foundation is to support arthritis research and to improve the quality of life for those affected by arthritis and related conditions. Planned giving is an important part of fulfilling this mission. The Foundation's planned giving department offers a wide variety of gift planning options, including estate gifts and gifts that provide donors with lifetime income.

We hope you decide to include a gift to the Arthritis Foundation in your will. Your greatest benefit from doing so will be the personal satisfaction of making a difference in the struggle against arthritis and related conditions. For more information on giving opportunities, call the Arthritis Foundation's planned giving department at 404/872-7100.

Ehlers-Danlos National Foundation
6399 Wilshire Blvd
Suite 510
Los Angeles, CA 90048
Tel: 323/651-3038
Fax: 323/651-1366
Web site: http://www.ednf.org
E-mail: ednfboard@aol.com

Fibromyalgia Alliance of America
P.O. Box 21990
Columbus, OH 43221-0980
Tel: 614/457-4222
Fax: 614/457-2729

Fibromyalgia Association of Greater
Washington, Inc.
13203 Valley Drive
Woodbridge, VA 22191-1531
Tel: 703/790-2324
Fax: 703/494-4103
Web site: http://www.fmagw.org

National Fibromyalgia Research
Association
P.O. Box 500
Salem, OR 97308
Tel: 503/588-1411
    800/574-3468
Fax: 503/315-7212
Web site: http://www.teleport.com/~nfra

Lupus Foundation of America
1300 Piccard Drive
Suite 200
Rockville, MD 20850-4303
Tel: 301/670-9292
    888/38-LUPUS
Fax: 301/670-9486
Web site: http://www.lupus.org

Lyme Disease Foundation
1 Financial Plaza
Hartford, CT 06103
Tel: 860/525-2000
    860/525-TICK
Fax: 860/525-8425
Web site: http://www.lyme.org

National Marfan Foundation
382 Main Street
Port Washington, NY 11050
Tel: 516/883-8712
    800/862-7326
Fax: 516/883-8040
Web site: http://www.marfan.org
E-mail: staff@marfan.org

The Paget Foundation
120 Wall Street, Suite 1602
New York, NY 10005
Tel: 212/509-5335
Fax: 212/509-8492
Web site: http://www.paget.org
E-mail: pagetfdn@aol.com

Reflex Sympathetic Dystrophy
Syndrome Association
116 Haddon Ave., Suite D
Haddonfield, NJ 08033
Tel: 609/795-8845
Fax: 609/795-8845
Web site: http://www.rsds.org
E-mail:jwbroatch@aol.com

Scleroderma Foundation
89 Newberry Street
Suite 201
Danvers, MA 01923-1075
Tel: 978/750-4499
    800/722-HOPE
Fax: 978/750-9902
Web site: http://www.scleroderma.org
E-mail:sfinfo@scleroderma.org

Scleroderma Research Foundation
2320 Bath Street
Suite 315
Santa Barbara, CA 93105
Tel: 805/563-9133
    800/441-2873
Fax: 805/563-2402
Web site: http://www.srfcure.org

Sjögren's Syndrome Foundation, Inc.
333 North Broadway
Suite 2000
Jericho, NY 11753
Tel: 516/933-6365
    800/475-6473
Fax: 516/933-6368
Web site: http://www.sjogrens.com
E-mail:ssf@idt.net

National Sjögren's Syndrome Association
P.O. Box 22066
Beachwood, OH 44122
Tel: 216/292-3866
    800/292-3877
Fax: 216/292-4955
Web site: http://www.sjogrens.org
E-mail: nssa@aol.com

Spondylitis Association of America
P.O. Box 5872
Sherman Oaks, CA 91413
Tel: 818/981-1616
    800/777-8189
Fax: 818/981-9826
Web site: http://www.spondylitis.org
E-mail: info@spondylitis.org

Index

Index

Index

Index

Index

Index

echinacea contraindicated
with, 208
fasting for, 164, 166
fish oil for, 209
folic acid and, 233
foods and, 162
ginger for, 214
GLA for, 212–213
green tea and, 219
homeopathy for, 49
intercessory prayer for, 93
LELL therapy for, 152
manipulation and, 44
massage for, 130
mind-body therapies for, 59
movement education programs
for, 99, 113
MSM for, 223
naturopathic medicine for, 39
oil supplements for, 172–173
qi gong for, 107
reflexology therapy and, 120
relaxation techniques for, 81–83
selenium for, 226
stress reduction programs for, 86
Swedish massage for, 122
tai chi chuan for, 107, 109
turmeric and, 229
vegan diet and, 168
vitamin B5 for, 232
weight loss and, 161
writing therapy for, 60
zinc sulfate for, 234
rheumatologists. See doctors
Rolfing techniques, 125

S
S-adenosylmethionine (SAM),
224–225
salai guggal. See boswellia
salesclerks, supplement advice
by, 179
SAM (S-adenosylmethionine),
224–225. See also folic acid
SAMe. See SAM
Sanskrit, herb names in, 192
scientific evidence. See also specific therapies

evaluating therapies using, 14–16
references for, 252–266
scientific research. See also clinical
trials
alternative therapies and, 4
arthritis in, 248–249
scleroderma
biofeedback and, 69
DHEA for, 205
DMSO for, 207
Scleroderma Foundation, 271
Scleroderma Research Foundation,
272
search services, professional, 17–18
sedatives, valerian, 230
seizure medications, acupuncture
and, 144
selenium, 226
Self-Help Course, arthritis, 55, 57
self-image, visualization for, 71, 74
sexual activity
acupuncture and, 144
therapist and, 10
Shanghai Institute, green tea study
by, 219
shark cartilage. See collagen
shiatsu, Japanese, 122–123, 138
shoulder pain, acupressure for, 139
Siberian ginseng (Eleutherococcus
senticosus), 216–217
side effects. See specific remedies
Sjogren's syndrome, acupuncture
and, 140
Sjogren's Syndrome Foundation,
Inc., 272
skin problems, 132. See also psoriasis
skinrolling massage, 123
smoking cessation, and spirituality,
91
soft tissue injuries, LELL therapy for,
152
Solanaceae (tomatoes). See diet,
nightshade-free
soybean/avocado oil, 191–192
spinal manipulation. See manipulation
spirituality

and health, 90–95
references for, 255
resources for, 92
Spondylitis Association of
America, 272
spondyloarthropathy, acupuncture
and, 140–141
sprains and strains, LELL therapy
for, 152
spray and stretch technique, 123
Stanford Arthritis Center, 55
steroids
acupuncture and, 144
aloe with, 190
CMO with, 200
dairy-free diet and, 167
DHEA with, 205
echinacea contraindicated with,
208
exercise and, 99
ginseng with, 217
zinc sulfate, 235
stiffness
See also charts, 7, 188–189
complementary therapies for, 7
glucosamine for, 217
homeopathy for, 49
massage for, 130
movement education programs
for, 111–115
reflexology therapy and, 120
selenium for, 226
supplements for, 188–189
vitamin B5 for, 232
zinc sulfate for, 234
stimulants, ginseng, 217
stinging nettle (Urtica dioica),
227–228
sting kit, for bee therapy, 150
St. John's wort (Hypericum perfora-
tum), 225–226
ginseng with, 217
study of, extensive, 177
stress, 54–58
biofeedback for, 68–69
bodywork for, 122, 130
Chinese medicine for, 35
diseases of, 54–61

Index

urinary tract infections, echinacea for, 208
Urtica dioica (stinging nettle), 227–228
"urtication," 227

V

valerian (*Valeriana officinalis*), 230
varicose veins, caution for, 132
Vedas (Hindu texts), 29
vegan diet, 170
vegetarian diet
  for arthritis, 162, 168, 170
  in ayurveda, 29–30
visualization, 56, 71–74
  conventional medicine with, 73
  references for, 253–254
  resources for, 73
vital life energy force
  prana, 29
  qi, 33
vitamin A (beta carotene), 210, 231
vitamin B, types of, 232
vitamin C, 177, 232
vitamin D, 210, 233
vitamin E, 233
vitamin supplements, 231–233. *See also* dietary supplements
  in chiropractic, 44
  for special diets, 161
  in vegan diet, 168
  in vegetarian diet, 170

W

water intake
  bodywork and, 124
  gout and, 169
Web sites. *See also specific therapies*
  alternative therapies, 17
  recommended, 251
weight, joint damage and, 161
Western energy therapies, 125–126
Western medicine
  alternative therapies with, 28
  chronic illnesses and, 3
  defined, 4–5

Wilson's disease, copper with, 204
World Health Foundation in Sedona, research services of, 18
World Health Organization, 140
wound healing
  aloe for, 190–191
  echinacea for, 208
writing therapy
  resources for, 60
  for rheumatoid arthritis, 60

X

X-rays, chiropractic and, 46

Y

Yale University, PEMF research by, 157
yam, wild (*Dioscorea villosa*)
  claims for, 234
  DHEA in, 205
yin and yang, Chinese, 33
yoga, 100–106
  ayurvedic, 29–30, 100
  breathing techniques in, 78
  gentle movements in, 98
  illustrated exercises of, 102–103
  meditation in, 62
  references for, 256
  resources for, 104–105
  stress reduction programs with, 85

Z

Zen Buddhism, meditation in, 62
Zen diet, 162
zinc sulfate, 234–235
Zingiber officinale (ginger), 214–215

STOCK PHOTO CREDITS

© Cotten Alston/Aristock, 52

© Terry Greene Photography, 26, 234

© Charles Gupton/Tony Stone, 8

© McGinnis Leathers/Aristock, 88

© Doug Plummer/Photonica, cover

© Patrick Ramsey/International Stock, 62, 253

© George Shelley/Stock Market, 98, 252

© Jamey Stillings/Tony Stone, 96

© Arthur Tilley/FPG, 72

© Jerome Tisne/Tony Stone, 127

© Greg Voight/International Stock, 44

© Cameron Wood Photography, 134, 160

© Caroline Wood/International Stock, 116

STOCK ILLUSTRATION CREDITS

© Jose Ortega, 11

© Mark Stearney, 71

MORE GREAT BOOKS FROM THE ARTHRITIS FOUNDATION!

Health Organizer: A Personal Health-Care Record
Keep your medical and insurance records in one easy-to-find location, and track your symptoms with useful prompts in this spiral-bound, tabbed organizer.
144 pages
#835-207
$11.95

Toward Healthy Living: A Wellness Journal
This beautifully designed, spiral-bound journal contains inspirational quotes and pain and mood charts that help you track the progress of your health.
144 pages
#835-205
$9.95

250 Tips for Making Live with Arthritis Easier
Packed with simple ideas for making daily tasks easier on your joints and less fatiguing, this book gives you ideas that you can start using today!
88 pages
#835-202
$9.95

Arthritis 101: Questions You Have. Answers You Need.
Get the fundamental text that gives you concise, easy-to-understand answers to even your most basic questions.
144 pages
#835-201
$11.95

Your Personal Guide to Living Well with Fibromyalgia
This hands-on workbook gives you the tools you need to take control over your condition and start down the path toward wellness.
224 pages
#835-203
$14.95

Primer on the Rheumatic Diseases, 11th Edition
This highly technical text was originally written for medical professionals and contains the latest information on the science, diagnosis and treatments for most rheumatic conditions.
516 pages
#750-3250
$39.95

Raising a Child with Arthritis: A Parent's Guide
This essential guide to understanding and coping with the challenges of childhood arthritis gives you reliable advice and information from top pediatric health professionals.
194 pages
#835-209
$14.95

Beyond Chaos: One Man's Journey Alongside His Chronically Ill Wife
Discover how living with his wife's chronic illness brought a new level of trust and intimacy to author Gregg Piburn's marriage, and let his experiences guide you through your own journey.
346 pages
#835-214
$14.95

Help Yourself: Recipes and Resources from the Arthritis Foundation
This limited-edition cookbook contains nearly 250 healthy recipes that are easy to prepare as well as information on special devices that simplify food preparation.
158 pages
#835-204
ONLY $12.95

PLACE YOUR ORDER TODAY!
1-800-207-8633
Operators are available to take your order
Monday – Friday, 8 a.m. – 6 p.m. EST

SOURCE CODE: ALTPAGE